Paediatric Symptom and Sign Sorter
Second Edition

Pediatric Diagnosis and Management

Pediatric Neurology, Second Edition
James F. Bale Jr., Joshua L. Bonkowsky, Francis M. Filloux, Gary L. Hedlund, Paul D. Larsen and Denise C. Morita

Pediatric Nail Disorders, First Edition
Robert Baran, Smail Hadj-Rabia, Robert Silverman

Pediatric Hair Disorders: An Atlas and Text, Third Edition
Juan Ferrando, Ramon Grimalt

Learning from Paediatric Patient Journeys: What Children and Their Families Can Tell Us, First Edition
Chloe Macaulay, Polly Powell, Caroline Fertleman

Great Ormond Street Handbook of Paediatrics, Second Edition
Stephan Strobel, Lewis Spitz, Stephen D. Marks

Paediatric Symptom Sorter, First Edition
Sahib El-Radhi

For more information about this series please visit: https://www.crcpress.com/Pediatric-Diagnosis-and-Management/book-series/CRCPEDDIAMAN

Paediatric Symptom and Sign Sorter
Second Edition

A. Sahib El-Radhi, MRCPCH, PhD, DCH
Harley Street Children's Clinic
Honorary Consultant Paediatrician, Queen Mary's Hospital, Sidcup
Honorary Senior Lecturer, Guy's and St Thomas'
School of Medicine, London, UK

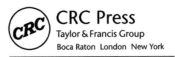

CRC Press
Taylor & Francis Group
Boca Raton London New York

CRC Press is an imprint of the
Taylor & Francis Group, an **informa** business

CRC Press
Taylor & Francis Group
6000 Broken Sound Parkway NW, Suite 300
Boca Raton, FL 33487-2742

International Standard Book Number-13: 978-1-138-31752-9 (Paperback)
978-1-138-31754-3 (Hardback)

Library of Congress Cataloging-in-Publication Data

Names: El-Radhi, A. Sahib., author.
Title: Paediatric symptom and sign sorter / by A Sahib El-Radhi.
Other titles: Paediatric symptom sorter | Pediatric diagnosis and management.
Description: Second edition. | Boca Raton, FL : CRC Press, Taylor & Francis Group, [2019] |
Series: Pediatric diagnosis and management | Preceded by Paediatric symptom sorter /
A. Sahib El-Radhi ; foreword by James Carroll. 2011. | Includes bibliographical references and index.
Identifiers: LCCN 2018047997| ISBN 9781138317543 (hardback : alk. paper) | ISBN 9781138317529
(pbk. : alk. paper) | ISBN 9780429455155 (ebook)
Subjects: | MESH: Diagnosis | Child | Signs and Symptoms | Diagnosis, Differential | Diagnostic
Techniques and Procedures | Infant | Handbooks
Classification: LCC RJ48 | NLM WS 39 | DDC 618.92/0075--dc23
LC record available at https://lccn.loc.gov/2018047997

Visit the Taylor & Francis Web site at
http://www.taylorandfrancis.com

and the CRC Press Web site at
http://www.crcpress.com

CONTENTS

AUTHOR

Dr A. Sahib El-Radhi was born and raised in Baghdad, Iraq where he attended primary and secondary schools. Then he attended the Medical School of the Free University of Berlin/Germany where he obtained the Bachelor's degree and later Ph.D.

For nearly 40 years, Dr El-Radhi has had the opportunity to work in many countries, including Germany, Kuwait, Iraq, Finland, and England, thereby gaining a wide experience on tropical infectious diseases and all kinds of interesting paediatric diseases.

Between 1993 and 2006, Dr El-Radhi was working as a consultant paediatrician at the University Queen Mary's Hospital Sidcup, Kent, England. He received the honour of senior honorary lecturer from the Medical School, London. He was involved in under- and postgraduate teaching for over 10 years and became the undergraduate tutor at the hospital. He was involved in research including numerous randomised controlled trials. His special interest has been fever-related diseases.

Dr El-Radhi has been MRCPCH and DCH examiner for nearly 20 years for our Royal College of paediatrics and child health. He has been a fellow of the Royal College of Paediatrics and Child Health since 1994. He has been a peer-reviewer of articles submitted to the Archives of Disease in Childhood, British Journal of Nursing and World Journal of Clinical Pediatrics, USA, where he is an editor as well. He has special interest in all scientific papers related to fever and has published two books on this subject.

1. Fever in Paediatric Practice by AS El-Radhi, James Carroll. Blackwell Scientific Publications, 1994. (translated to Russian language).
2. Clinical Manual of Fever in Children by AS El-Radhi, J Carroll, N Klein. Springer Publication 2009. (translated to Spanish language).
3. Essential Paediatrics in Primary Care by AS El-Radhi, S Gregson, N Paul, A Rahman. Radcliffe Publishers 2011.
4. Paediatric Symptoms Sorter by AS El-Radhi. Radcliffe Publishers 2011.
5. Asthma by AS El-Radhi. MacMillan Publisher 2011.
6. Clinical Manual of Fever in Children by AS El-Radhi, 2nd ed. Springer Pub. 2018.
7. Paediatric Symptoms and Signs Sorter by AS El-Radhi. CRC Press.

Currently he is a part-time paediatrician at the BMI Chelsfield Park Hospital, Kent, England. He has now more time to focus on his special interest that is searching medical journals and Internet for scientific publications and writing medical books and articles. In 2017, he was pleased to publish 8 papers in medical journals. In 2018, he wrote two books. In 2019, he already signed a contract to write a new book on Avoiding Misdiagnosis in Paediatric Practice. He submitted a proposal with an American colleague, Professor Park to write a pediatric-neurological book on Pediatric Neuro-inflammatory Diseases. In addition, Dr El-Radhi is engaging in his free time with charity organisations and playing tennis.

INTRODUCTION

When I reached an agreement with the publisher to write a second edition of my book *Paediatric Symptom Sorter*, I was very pleased. After a seven-to-eight-year period since the publication of the first edition, a huge bulk of literature had accumulated that needed to be incorporated in a new edition and transmitted to the potential readers of the book. In addition, the text of the first edition was due for improvement. As I indicated in the first edition, there was a minor and occasional difficulty regarding what to label 'Common' versus 'Rare' and which diagnoses should belong to 'Children' and which to 'Infants'. Additionally, under 'Top Tips' and 'Red Flags', one could argue that some statements appearing under one heading may have been more appropriately placed under the other. It is hoped that this difficulty has been overcome in this second edition; and with more clinical experience in paediatric practice and critical judgement, I am pleased to say that I believe an improved text has been achieved. This second edition, now titled *Paediatric Symptom and Sign Sorter*, constitutes a major revision and reorganization of the text based on a complete review of the field of paediatrics. There is a new chapter and many new sections, as well as substantial modification and expansion compared to the first edition. Colour photographs (supplied by Shutterstock.com) have also been added to illustrate common clinical presentations.

The publication of the second edition coincides with recent publications of significant advances in the literature related to the subjects of this book. Knowledge of the majority of the topics has expanded. Accordingly, every area of the new edition has been carefully scrutinized for possible improvement that included these recent advances. The whole text has been updated and every statement has been subject to careful consideration. It is hoped that accuracy and scientific evidence have prevailed in every section of the book, which came as a result of long personal paediatric experience and repeated revision, backed up by a thorough search of the literature. Diagnosis is on the best available evidence, and established guidelines have been included wherever available and appropriate. However, it is not possible to cover all health issues arising in detail, so the end of each section has references that should be consulted when more information is needed and desired.

The vast majority of paediatric books on the market are system-based, starting with a chapter such as upper respiratory infections and ending up with another chapter such as neurology. However, children present with a plethora of symptoms; therefore, using the traditional paediatric textbook to reach the right diagnosis is difficult and sometimes impossible. It is hoped that this symptom-based book will aid the clinician to reach the correct diagnosis easily and quickly. It has been written for all professionals who deal with sick children, including junior and senior paediatricians, primary care doctors, and particularly those who need rapid reference, such as doctors on call. Paediatric nurses, with their increasing role in managing sick children, may use this book as reference in their clinical activity. Medical students on the paediatric wards or in the A&E department may also use this book for discussions with their more qualified colleagues.

In our continuing effort, we tried to address as many topics as possible that are related to the health and welfare of children and youth. Our goal, as in the previous edition, is to provide information that will help the professionals dealing with children to provide better care. It is hoped the information inside the book will add to the knowledge of clinicians who will apply this information to reach a swift diagnosis. Once a diagnosis is established, children are ultimately the beneficiaries by getting the necessary help because their complaints have been solved.

LIST OF ABBREVIATIONS

A&E	Accident and emergency
AAP	Acute abdominal pain
ACS	Acute confusional state
AD	Atopic dermatitis
ADH	Antidiuretic hormone
ADHD	Attention deficit hyperactivity disorder
AED	Anti-epileptic drug
AHG	Acute herpetic gingivostomatitis
ANA	Anti-nuclear antibodies
ANUG	Acute necrotising ulcerative gingivitis
AOS	Arterial oxygen saturation
AR	Allergic rhinitis
ARF	Acute renal failure
ASO	Antistreptolysin O
AVM	Arteriovenous malformation
AVP	Arginine vasopressin
BC	Blood culture
BG	Blood glucose
BMI	Body mass index
BPPV	Benign paroxysmal positional vertigo
BPVC	Benign paroxysmal vertigo of childhood
CAH	Congenital adrenal hyperplasia
CANOMAD	Chronic ataxic neuropathy with ophthalmoplegia, M-protein, agglutination and disialosyl antibodies
CCF	Congestive cardiac failure
CCMT	Congenital cutis marmorata telangiectasia
CD	Crohn's disease
CF	Cystic fibrosis
CFS	Chronic fatigue syndrome
CHARGE	Coloboma, heart defect, atresia rate of the choanae, retarded growth, genital hypoplasia and ear anomaly
CHD	Congenital heart disease
CMA	Chromosomal microarray
CMN	Congenital melanocytic naevi
CMV	Cytomegalovirus
CNS	Central nervous system
CO	Carbon monoxide
CP	Cerebral palsy
CPK	Creatine phosphokinase
CREST	Calcinosis, Raynaud's phenomenon, oesophageal dysmotility, sclerodactyly and telangiectasia
CRF	Chronic renal failure
CRP	C-reactive protein
CSF	Cerebrospinal fluid
CT	Computed tomography
CTD	Connective tissue disease
CULLP	Congenital unilateral lower lip palsy

CV	Cyclic vomiting
CVS	Congenital varicella syndrome
DHEA	Dehydroepiandrosterone
DHEAS	Dehydroepiandrosterone sulfate
DI	Diabetes insipidus
DIC	Disseminated intravascular coagulation
DKA	Diabetic ketoacidosis
DM	Diabetes mellitus
DMD	Duchenne muscular dystrophy
DP	Delayed puberty
DV	Dysfunctional voiding
EBV	Epstein–Barr virus
ECC	Early childhood caries
ECG	Electrocardiogram
EEG	Electroencephalogram
EKC	Epidemic keratoconjunctivitis
EM	Erythema multiforme
EMG	Electromyogram
EMLA	Eutectic mixture of local anaesthetics
ENT	Ear, nose and throat
EOAE	Evoked otoacoustic emissions
ESR	Erythrocyte sedimentation rate
ET	Essential tremor
ETN	Erythema toxicum neonatorum
FB	Foreign body
FBC	Full blood count
FCUS	Familial cold urticaria syndrome
FGID	Functional gastrointestinal disorder
FHH	Functional hypo-gonadotropic hypogonadism
FMF	Familial Mediterranean fever
FS	Febrile seizure
FSH	Follicle-stimulating hormone
FTT	Failure to thrive
FWF	Fever without focus
GAHS	Group A β-haemolytic streptococci
GAS	Group A streptococci
GBS	Guillain–Barré syndrome
GE	Gastroenteritis
GF	Glandular fever
GH	Growth hormone
GI	Gastrointestinal
GIB	Gastrointestinal bleeding
GN	Glomerulonephritis
GnRH	Gonadotropin-releasing hormone
GO	Gastro-oesophageal
HAE	Hereditary angioedema
HAV	Hepatitis A virus
Hb	Haemoglobin
HbA2	Haemoglobin α-2
HbF	Haemoglobin F
HbS	Haemoglobin S

HD	Hirschsprung's disease
HDN	Haemorrhagic disease of the newborn
HHS	Hyperglycaemia hyperosmolar state
HHT	Hereditary haemorrhagic telangiectasia
HHV-6	Human herpesvirus 6
HIDS	Hyperimmunoglobulinemia D syndrome
HIE	Hypoxic-ischaemic encephalopathy
HIV	Human immunodeficiency virus
HL	Hodgkin's lymphoma
HPV	Human papillomavirus
HRCT	High-resolution computed tomography
HSP	Henoch–Schönlein purpura
HSV	Herpes simplex virus
HUS	Haemolytic-uraemic syndrome
HVA	Homovanillic acid
HVDRR	Hereditary vitamin D-resistant rickets
IBD	Inflammatory bowel disease
IBS	Irritable bowel syndrome
ICP	Intracranial pressure
ID	Intellectual disability
IDA	Iron-deficiency anaemia
IgM-RF	Immunoglobulin M rheumatoid factor
IH	Inguinal hernia
IHB	Indirect hyperbilirubinaemia
IQ	Intelligence quotient
ISO	Idiopathic scrotal oedema
ITP	Idiopathic thrombocytopenic purpura
IV	Intravenous
JDM	Juvenile dermatomyositis
JIA	Juvenile idiopathic arthritis
JRA	Juvenile rheumatoid arthritis
KLS	Kleine–Levin syndrome
LAMB	A syndrome of lentigines, atrial myxoma, mucocutaneous myxoma and blue naevi
LEOPARD	A syndrome of lentigines, ECG abnormalities, ocular hypertelorism, pulmonary stenosis, abnormal genitalia, retarded growth and deafness
LFT	Liver function tests
LH	Luteinising hormone
LMN	Lower motor neurone
LP	Lumbar puncture
LRTI	Lower respiratory tract infection
MA	Mesenteric adenitis
MCD	Meningococcal disease
MCH	Mean corpuscular haemoglobin
MCS	Meningococcal septicaemia
MCV	Mean cell volume
MELAS	Mitochondrial encephalopathy, lactic acidosis and stroke-like episodes
MG	Myasthenia gravis
MRI	Magnetic resonance imaging
MSE	Monosymptomatic enuresis
MSPS	Musculoskeletal pain syndrome
MWS	Muckle–Wells syndrome

MWT	Mallory–Weiss tear
NAI	Non-accidental injury
NCSE	Non-convulsive status epilepticus
NDI	Nephrogenic diabetes insipidus
NE	Nocturnal enuresis
NEC	Necrotising enterocolitis
NF-1	Neurofibromatosis type 1
NFLE	Nocturnal frontal lobe epilepsy
NIDDM	Non-insulin-dependent diabetes mellitus
NMD	Neuromuscular disease
NMSE	Non-monosymptomatic enuresis
NREM	Non-rapid eye movement
NS	Nephrotic syndrome
NSAID	Non-steroidal anti-inflammatory drug
NUG	Necrotising ulcerative gingivostomatitis
NV	Neonatal varicella
OAB	Overactive bladder
OCD	Obsessive-compulsive disorder
OE	Otitis externa
OM	Otitis media
OME	Otitis media with effusion
ORS	Oral rehydration solution
OSA	Obstructive sleep apnoea
OTC	Over-the-counter
OTCD	Ornithine transcarbamylase deficiency
PBB	Protracted bacterial bronchitis
PCOS	Polycystic ovary syndrome
PCR	Polymerase chain reaction
PF	Periodic fever
PFAPA	Periodic fever, aphthous stomatitis, pharyngitis and cervical adenitis
PHACE	Posterior fossa brain malformation, haemangioma, arterial lesions, cardiac and eye abnormalities
PHN	Post-herpetic neuralgia
PID	Pelvic inflammatory disease
PIH	Post-inflammatory hyperpigmentation
PLMD	Periodic limb movement disorder
PNE	Primary nocturnal enuresis
POS	Polycystic ovary syndrome
POTS	Postural tachycardia syndrome
PP	Precocious puberty
PPP	Partial precocious puberty
PS	Pyloric stenosis
PSGN	Poststreptococcal glomerulonephritis
PT	Prothrombin time
PTT	Partial thromboplastin time
PUO	Pyrexia of unknown origin
RAP	Recurrent abdominal pain
RAST	Radioallergosorbent test
RBC	Red blood cell
RBC/HPF	Red blood cells per high-power field
RDS	Respiratory distress syndrome

RE	Rectal examination
ReA	Reactive arthritis
ReF	Relapsing fever
REM	Rapid eye movement
RF	Rheumatic fever
RFT	Renal function tests
RhF	Rheumatoid factor
ROP	Retinopathy of prematurity
RP	Rectal prolapse
RSV	Respiratory syncytial virus
RTA	Renal tubular acidosis
SA	Septic arthritis
SCA	Sickle-cell anaemia
SCBU	Special care baby unit
SCD	Sudden cardiac death
SCFE	Slipped capital femoral epiphysis
SD	Seborrhoeic dermatitis
SE	Status epilepticus
SHH	Structural hypo-gonadotropic hypogonadism
SLE	Systemic lupus erythematosus
SMA	Spinal muscular atrophy
SNE	Secondary nocturnal enuresis
SS	Short stature
ST	Sinus tachycardia
STD	Sexually transmitted disease
SVT	Supraventricular tachycardia
T1D	Type 1 diabetes
TAR	Thrombocytopenia-absent radius
TB	Tuberculosis
TC	Tinea capitis
TDC	Thyroglossal duct cyst
TFT	Thyroid function test
TORCH	Toxoplasmosis, rubella, cytomegalovirus and herpes
TRAPS	TNF-receptor associated periodic syndrome
U&E	Urea and electrolytes
UGIB	Upper gastrointestinal bleeding
UMN	Upper motor neurone
URTI	Upper respiratory tract infection
UTI	Urinary tract infection
VD	Vaginal discharge
VMA	Vanillylmandelic acid
VN	Vestibular nerve
VR	Vasomotor rhinitis
VSC	Volatile sulphur compound
VSD	Ventricular septal defect
VT	Ventricular tachycardia
WBC	White blood cell
WPW	Wolff–Parkinson–White

1 CHEST

ACUTE SHORTNESS OF BREATH (DYSPNOEA)

Clinical Overview

Dyspnoea is a subjective feeling of difficulty in breathing. Children or parents may describe dyspnoea as 'getting easily tired' or 'can't keep up with other kids'. It may occur spontaneously or during certain activities such as exercise or during feeding in infants. Dyspnoea is a common symptom of a variety of cardio-pulmonary diseases. Respiratory diseases, such as asthma, remain the most common reason for dyspnoea. In older children, psychological factors can contribute to the sensation of dyspnoea. Congestive cardiac failure (CCF) is an important cause of dyspnoea at any age of childhood. Children presenting with dyspnoea usually have other symptoms and signs of respiratory distress syndrome, including tachypnoea, subcostal recession, tachycardia and chest tightness. The term may also include 'unusual pattern of breathing'. For example, hyperpnoea, which occurs in metabolic acidosis, such as diabetic ketoacidosis, may also give a sensation of dyspnoea.

Possible Diagnoses

Onset in Infants	Children
Common	
Respiratory distress syndrome	Asthma
Transient tachypnoea	Viral-induced wheeze
Viral-induced wheeze	Pneumonia
Bronchiolitis	CCF
CCF	Psychogenic
Rare	
Pulmonary oedema	Pulmonary oedema
Pneumonia	Obstructive airway diseases
Pneumothorax	Pulmonary embolism
Persistent pulmonary hypertension	Inhaled foreign body
Pleural effusion	Chronic lung disease
Pulmonary hypoplasia	Neuromuscular disease (e.g. myasthenia gravis)
Pericardial tamponade	Hyperventilation
	Pulmonary embolism

Differential Diagnosis at a Glance

	Asthma	Viral-Induced	Pneumonia	Cardiac Failure	Psychogenic
Grunting	No	No	Yes	No	No
Tachypnoea	Yes	Yes	Yes	Yes	No
Wheeze	Yes	Yes	No	Possible	No
Fever	Possible	Possible	Yes	No	No
Reduced peak flow	Yes	Possible	Possible	Possible	No

Recommended Investigations

Oxygen saturation monitoring (oximetry), peak flow measurements and, in severe cases, the following:

*** Blood gas measurements are essential frontline investigations
*** Lung function tests can differentiate between obstructive and restrictive causes of dyspnoea
*** A chest X-ray may show hyperinflation (asthma); consolidation (pneumonia); pneumothorax
*** Echocardiography and electrocardiogram (ECG) in patients with suspected heart disease

Top Tips

- A clear distinction between bronchiolitis and bronchitis in the first 2 years of life is difficult and is of no therapeutic significance.
- The history of a child with shortness of breath is incomplete without asking about symptoms associated with activities such as running or bike riding or exposure to cooler weather.
- Dyspnoea during exercise is frequently caused by asthma. Peak flow measurements before and after the exercise help to establish the diagnosis. Observing the child using the inhaler is essential.
- Wheezing is not a symptom of pneumonia, while grunting with flaring of alae nasi is a symptom.
- The differentiation between cardiac and pulmonary causes of dyspnoea can be difficult. The presence of a murmur, liver enlargement and relative tachycardia favour cardiac causes.
- An aid to differentiate cardiac from pulmonary dyspnoea is the hyperbaric oxygen test by breathing 100%. In pulmonary diseases there will be a normalisation of the oxygen saturation.
- The question whether to admit a child with asthma can be difficult. If oxygen saturation in air is greater than 95% and peak flow measurement greater than 70% of the expected, he/she can be managed with medications at home.
- Regular physical activity by a child with asthma is associated with an improvement of disease control and life quality. Parents often restrain their asthmatic children from engaging in physical activity for unfounded fear of asthma exacerbation.
- When an adolescent presents with hyperventilation, ask about other psychosomatic complaints, e.g. any problem with swallowing difficulty suggestive of 'globus hystericus'.

Red Flags

- An asthmatic child who suddenly becomes dyspnoeic, with retrosternal pain, may not always have exacerbation of asthma. Pneumothorax or pneumomediastinum should be considered. Pneumomediastinum is caused by alveolar rupture, leading to air infiltration along the bronchiolar sheath with air reaching the mediastinum. Computed tomography (CT) scan is the golden standard to diagnose it.
- An infant with no murmur detected at birth but a murmur at the age of 6 weeks is likely to be due to ventricular septal defect (VSD). This infant may soon develop CCF if the VSD is large.
- Asthma can have some shadows in the chest X-ray; these do not indicate pneumonia and will disappear with anti-asthmatic treatment, and antibiotics are not indicated.
- An infant with prolonged feeding time, who requires rest periods during feeding, or who displays breathlessness while feeding can have an underlying cardiac failure.
- Remember that oxygen saturations represent the oxygenated haemoglobin (Hb) to the total Hb, so oxygen saturation can still be normal in the presence of anaemia or carbon monoxide poisoning.

FURTHER READING

McCarter T. Asthma – The national surveillance data and the national asthma education and prevention program's expert panel report 3. *Am Health Drug Benefits* 2008;1(2):35–50.

BREAST ENLARGEMENT IN BOYS (GYNAECOMASTIA)

Clinical Overview

Gynaecomastia is the most common disease of the male breast. It is defined as a benign diffuse enlargement of the breast due to the presence of mammary tissue, mainly glandular proliferation, in the male. It is the result of oestrogen-androgen imbalance (whether an increase in oestrogen production, a relative decrease of testosterone production or a combination of both). In the male, androgens are important in inhibiting stimulatory oestrogenic effects on breast tissue. Gynaecomastia has two peaks: in the neonatal period, with an occurrence of 60%–90% of babies, and a second peak occurring at puberty which is a common condition affecting the majority of male children and regressing spontaneously in 12–18 months. This type of gynaecomastia needs to be differentiated from obesity-related breast enlargement (pseudo-gynaecomastia), which is composed of adipose tissue (and not glandular tissue), medication-induced gynaecomastia, familial gynaecomastia and local lesions inside the breast such as tumour.

Possible Diagnoses

Infants	Children
Common	
Physiologic (maternal hormones)	Puberty (about two-thirds of all boys)
Infection	Drugs (exposure to oestrogen)
	Familial gynaecomastia (autosomal dominant)
	Klinefelter's syndrome
	Obesity
Rare	
	Benign mass (lipoma, cysts, haematoma)
	Testicular failure
	Growth hormone therapy
	Neurofibromatosis
	Congenital adrenogenital (11ß-hydroxylase deficiency)
	Adrenal tumour (feminising tumour)
	Hypogonadism and cryptorchidism
	Testicular tumour (Leydig cell tumour, usually benign)
	Hyperthyroidism
	Prolactinoma
	Liver tumours
	Liver cirrhosis
	Chronic renal failure
	Peutz–Jeghers' syndrome
	McCune–Albright's syndrome
	Breast carcinoma
	Androgen insensitivity syndrome
	Reifenstein's syndrome (hypogonadism)

Differential Diagnosis at a Glance

	Puberty	Drugs	Familial	Klinefelter Syndrome	Obesity
Learning difficulty	No	No	No	Yes	No
Hypogonadism	No	No	No	Yes	No
Unilateral	Possible	Possible	Possible	Possible	No
Noted at puberty	Yes	No	No	Yes	No
Spontaneous resolution	Yes	No	No	No	Possible

Recommended Investigations

In most cases, tests are not necessary. Some cases may need the following:

* ** Thyroid function tests to assess thyroid function
* ** Testosterone level for suspected hypogonadism
* ** Chromosomal analysis if Klinefelter's syndrome suspected
* ** 17-hydroxyprogesterone and other tests for congenital adrenogenital syndrome
* ** Ultrasound scan for breast evaluation (breast mass, renal and testicular tumours)
* ** Magnetic resonance imaging (MRI) for cerebral lesions (e.g. prolactinoma)
* ** Mammography to evaluate true gynaecomastia from benign or malignant tumours
* ** Biopsy for suspected testicular tumours

Top Tips

* Enlargement of the breasts occurs in most male and female neonates as a result of stimulation by maternal hormones. Spontaneous regression is the rule. Their families need to be reassured.
* During puberty, up to two-thirds of boys develop gynaecomastia that may be unilateral and tender. It usually begins at age 10–12 years and peaks at age 13–14 years, and regression is usual within 18 months.
* In gynaecomastia, a firm or rubbery mass of tissue can be felt extending symmetrically from the nipple. In obese boys the breasts are enlarged due to fat tissue accumulation (pseudo-gynaecomastia), without the characteristic rubbery consistency. Because of the increasing incidence of obesity, pseudo-gynaecomastia is increasing.
* The mean hormonal concentrations of follicle-stimulating hormone (FSH), luteinising hormone (LH), prolactin, testosterone and eostradiol in boys with gynaecomastia are the same as in boys without it.
* Drugs inducing gynaecomastia include ketoconazole, spironolactone, digoxin, methyldopa, marijuana and anti-ulcer (e.g. omeprazole) and antiretroviral drugs. They should be discontinued whenever possible. In a month after discontinuation, gynaecomastia should have regressed.
* Surgical removal of the enlarged breast is rarely indicated except for marked enlargement that has caused emotional stress to the child.

Red Flags

* In neonatal gynaecomastia, discharge from the nipple (colostrums) should not be squeezed or pressed to avoid infection. Although it usually regresses within 2–3 weeks of age, in some cases enlargement continues up to 6 months of age.

- In contrast to the common occurrence of pubertal gynaecomastia, pre-pubertal gynae-comastia is rare but often unrecognised. Although the majority of them are idiopathic, it could be a sign of serious underlying disorders. Full evaluation is required.
- In any child with gynaecomastia, effort should be made to exclude exposure to oestrogen, accidental or therapeutic. Increased pigmentation of the nipple and areola is an important clue.
- Gynaecomastia associated with neurological manifestations such as headaches and/or visual disturbance could be caused by pituitary tumour. A cranial MRI is urgently required.
- In a child with gynaecomastia, testes should be examined to exclude tumour or testicular failure.
- Any gynaecomastia with galactorrhoea (spontaneous flow of milk) may suggest the presence of prolactinoma as an underlying pathology; an urgent serum prolactin and cranial MRI are required.
- Gynaecomastia can later become fibrotic, firm, sometimes hard, and has to be differentiated from breast cancer, which is rare and accounts for less than 1% of cancers in men. Red flags include unilateral mass that is hard, fixed, peripheral to the nipple or associated with nipple discharge, skin changes or lymphadenopathy.
- Klinefelter's syndrome is common (1:500–1,000 of newborn males, making it the most common chromosomal aberration) and is associated with gynaecomastia in 80% of cases; the risk of breast cancer is 16 times higher than in other men. Monitoring the gynaecomastia is important.

FURTHER READING

Cuhaci N, Polaf SB, Evranos B et al. Gynecomastia: Clinical evaluation and management. *Indian J Endocrinol* 2014;18(2):150–158.

BREAST LUMPS

Clinical Overview

Breast development normally occurs in girls aged 8½ to 13½ years in five stages; development is not completed until late teens and early twenties. The vast majority of breast masses in children are usually benign and self-limited. Neonatal bilateral breast hypertrophy due to maternal hormonal influence is a very common finding in both sexes. Breast buds and thelarche may occur in female toddlers; the condition is usually benign if it occurs in isolation. Nonetheless, a lump in the breast is an alarming sign because parents associate any breast swelling with cancer. A thorough history and physical examination, sometimes requiring needle aspiration and biopsy, are essential in any child who has a mass in the breast.

Possible Diagnoses

Infants	Children
Common	
Bilateral breast enlargement	Thelarche (including premature thelarche)
Mastitis/abscess	Breast buds
Haemangioma	Precocious puberty cyst
Injury to the breast	Benign tumour (e.g. fibroadenoma haemangioma)
	Breast engorgement
Rare	
	Trauma
	Drugs (oestrogen, systemic or topical)
	Intramammary lymph node
	Malignant tumours (rhabdomyosarcoma, non-Hodgkin's lymphoma, metastatic neuroblastoma)
	Virginal hypertrophy (macromastia)
	Fibrocystic (mammary dysplasia)
	Lipoma
	Fat necrosis
	Macromastia

Differential Diagnosis at a Glance

	Thelarche	Breast Buds	Precocious Puberty	Benign Tumour	Breast Engorgement
Often unilateral	Yes	Yes	Possible	Yes	Possible
Adrenarche present	No	No	Yes	No	No
Growth spurt	No	Yes	Yes	Possible	Yes
Isolated round mass	No	Yes	No	Yes	Yes
May affect toddlers	Yes	Yes	Yes	Possible	No

Recommended Investigations

- *** Ultrasound scan to diagnose breast masses, e.g. a cyst or normal thelarche with normal tissue
- *** Pelvic ultrasonography for precocious puberty in girls

*** Fine-needle aspiration and guided biopsy are essential for evaluation of breast masses
*** Hormonal assay in blood (LH, FSH, sex hormones) for cases with precocious puberty
*** Cranial MRI may demonstrate a CNS abnormality in children with precious puberty
** Wrist X-ray for bone age to assess osseous maturation for cases of precocious puberty

Top Tips

- Premature breast development (thelarche) is defined as an isolated breast enlargement in girls before the age of 7 years. Precocious puberty in girls is defined by the presence of other puberty signs (pubic and/or axillary hair, growth spurt) before the age of 8 years in girls and before the age of 9 years in boys.
- Fibroadenoma, the most frequent breast tumour, occurs mostly in adolescents, which is usually solitary and benign.
- Breast trauma is common, resulting often from contact sport. Haematoma, contusion and fat necrosis may occur. The latter results from cystic changes or fibrosis within the breast.
- Painful engorgement of the breast (mastodynia) occurs physiologically in association with ovulatory cycles and pathologically in lactating mothers.
- In contrast to adults, mammography is not used in paediatrics because of the extremely low incidence of cancer and the risk of radiation, and because the dense breast tissue of adolescents obstructs adequate visualisation.

Red Flags

- Breast buds (stage 2 of breast development) heralding puberty in girls may be tender on palpation; this does not suggest inflammation.
- Although premature thelarche is a benign condition starting as early as under 1 year of age, thorough examination of the child is essential to ensure there are no signs of precocious puberty or pigmentation.
- The vast majority of breast masses can be diagnosed clinically or with the help of ultrasound scan. Only occasionally is fine-needle aspiration biopsy required; surgery is best avoided to prevent deformity.
- If cysts are suspected, these often vary in size in relation to the menstrual cycle, so a patient should be re-examined 2 weeks after the initial examination.
- Remember that a relapse of acute lymphoblastic leukaemia may present as a breast lump.
- Although malignant tumours are rare in children, their incidence is 2%–3% of all breast masses in adolescent girls. Early menarche in association anovulatory cycles is a risk factor.
- A breast cancer is recognised by its rapid growth; it is hard and not freely mobile. Changes of the overlying skin including ulceration and nipple discharges are worrying signs.

FURTHER READING

Kennedy RD, Boughey JC. Management of paediatric and adolescent breast masses. *Semin Plast Surg* 2013;27(1):19–22.

CHEST PAIN

Clinical Overview

Chest pain is a common complaint in children. It is the second most frequent cause of referral to paediatric cardiologists after cardiac murmur. Although chest pain in adults is considered a medical emergency because of possible associated heart attack, the overwhelming majority of children have a non-cardiac aetiology. The most common causes of chest pain include idiopathic, injury, musculoskeletal myalgia, pulmonary diseases (e.g. asthma), cardiac, gastrointestinal disorders and psychogenic causes. Many teenagers present with psychogenic chest pain, often with hyperventilation, reflecting anxiety generated by some events. Other teenagers have chest pain because of benign transient intercostal muscle spasm. Chest pain can be acute or chronic, which lasts by definition longer than 6 months. Although chronic or recurrent chest pain is likely to be benign (mostly caused by anxiety), this complaint often leads to numerous school absences, restriction of normal activities and considerable worry for patients and their parents.

Possible Diagnoses

Infants	Children
Common	
Inflammatory changes (cellulitis)	Idiopathic
Child abuse (e.g. rib fracture)	Psychogenic (anxiety or stress)
Trauma/injury	Costochondritis
Pneumonia	Direct trauma to the chest
Chest drain (therapeutic)	Pulmonary (pneumonia, asthma, pleurisy)
Rare	
Acute chest syndrome (sickle-cell anaemia [SCA])	Acid reflux
Anomalous origin of the coronary arteries	Myositis (such as dermatomyositis)
	Ischaemic heart disease (e.g. Kawasaki's disease)
Kawasaki's disease	Marfan's syndrome (because of dissecting aortic aneurysm)
Scurvy	Cardiac (e.g. aortic stenosis, pericarditis)
	SCA (causing ischaemic chest pain)
	Bornholm's disease
	Herpes zoster

Differential Diagnosis at a Glance

	Idiopathic	Psychogenic	Costochondritis	Trauma	Pulmonary
Abnormal physical findings	No	No	Yes	Possible	Yes
Previous episodes	Possible	Yes	No	No	Possible
>10 years of age	Possible	Yes	No	No	No
Antecedent viral upper respiratory tract infection (URTI)	No	No	Yes	No	Possible
Localised (non-diffuse)	Yes	No	Yes	Possible	Possible

Recommended Investigations

** Full blood count (FBC) may show anaemia in SCA

** Chest X-ray for cases of pericarditis, pneumonia, chest syndrome for SCA

*** ECG and 24-hour ECG monitoring if cardiac cases
** Exercise stress test for suspected cardiac diseases
*** Echocardiography for suspected cardiac disease
** Endoscopy if a gastric source of the pain is suspected (e.g. in gastro-oesophageal [GO] reflux)

Top Tips (Top Clues)

- The first clinical issue in a child with chest pain is to decide whether the history and clinical findings suggest an organic or non-organic cause.
- Idiopathic chest pain is the most common cause, occurring in 20%–45% of cases. It is defined by absence of cause for the chest pain after a thorough history, physical examination and laboratory testing, excluding thereby organic disease such as cardiac or pulmonary disease.
- Chest pain, discomfort or heaviness on exercise suggests exercise-induced bronchospasm. A bronchodilator before the exercise is likely to prevent these symptoms and suggest the diagnosis.
- Costochondritis (Tietze's syndrome), frequently caused by viral infection, is characterised by localised swelling of the costo-chondral, costo-sternal or sterno-clavicular joints, mostly involving the second and third ribs. Chest movements or taking a deep breath may worsen the pain.
- Acid reflux can cause retrosternal or left-sided chest pain with or without epigastric pain, often presenting as burning sensation.
- A typical psychogenic chest pain: dull or sharp, of short duration and unrelated to exercise. Teenagers are mostly affected. Inquire about loss of a relative, a pending examination, bullying at school, breakup in relations with a friend or a close relative who has had angina or a heart attack.
- Chronic or recurrent episodes of chest pain lasting more than 6 months without abnormal findings are likely to be psychogenic. This cause accounts for 5%–10% of cases, mostly in girls.

Red Flags

- Chest pain in infancy is difficult to diagnose. An infant who presents with sweating, restlessness and crying (as equivalent signs for expressing chest pain) may have a serious cardiac disease, e.g. acute chest syndrome in SCA or anomalous origin of the coronary arteries.
- Serious attention has to be given to children who present with abnormal physical examination findings, abnormal ECG, exertional chest pain (after excluding respiratory disease), associated palpitation or a family history of cardiomyopathy. Referral for further evaluation is essential.
- When the presentation of chest pain or discomfort is associated with syncope, a cardiac cause needs to be considered such as aortic stenosis, atrial myxoma (associated with tuberous sclerosis), hypertrophic cardiomyopathy, long Q-T syndrome and supraventricular tachycardia (SVT) with very rapid heart rate.
- Patients with marfanoid appearance and chest pain require close attention because they are at risk of dilatation of the ascending aorta and dissecting aneurysm.

FURTHER READING

Friedman KG, Alexander ME. Chest pain and syncope in children: A practical approach to the diagnosis of cardiac disease. *J Pediatr* 2013;163(3):896–901.

COUGH

Clinical Overview

Cough is one of the most common symptoms in children. It has been estimated that young children develop five to eight episodes of cough a year that typically resolve within 7–10 days. A viral URTI is the most common cause of acute cough, while asthma is the most common cause of chronic cough. Cough may be a symptom of extrapulmonary disease such as myocarditis or congestive cardiac failure. For practical purpose, cough is defined as acute (<2 weeks), or chronic (>4 weeks). Cough has to be persistent daily to be defined as chronic. Chronic cough is subdivided into specific (cough in the presence of identifiable respiratory disease or known cause) and non-specific cough (absence of respiratory disease or known cause). Cough is also divided into dry (e.g. asthma) and wet-moist (bronchiectasis). Prescribing medications to suppress the cough is not part of paediatric practice, but finding the underlying cause of cough is essential.

Possible Diagnoses

Onset in Infants	Children
Common	
URTI	URTI (e.g. viral URTI, croup)
Lower respiratory tract infection (LRTI)	LRTI (e.g. pneumonia, bronchitis)
Viral-induced wheeze	Asthma
Aspiration	Allergy (dust or pollen inhalation)
GO reflux	Psychogenic (Habit cough)
Rare	
Tracheo-oesophageal fistula	Ciliary dyskinesia
Bronchiectasis	Inhaled foreign body
Congenital lobar emphysema	Cystic fibrosis (CF)
Pertussis	Drugs (angiotensin-converting enzyme inhibitor)
	Pertussis
	Bronchiectasis
	α-1-Antitypic deficiency
	Drugs (angiotensin-converting enzyme inhibitors)
	Pulmonary tuberculosis
	Oesophageal-tracheal fistula
	Severe chest wall deformity
	Achalasia

Differential Diagnosis at a Glance

	URTI	LRTI	Asthma	Allergy	Psychogenic
Associated wheeze	No	Possible	Yes	Possible	No
The only symptom	No	No	No	Possible	Possible
Runny/blocked nose	Yes	No	Possible	Yes	No
Associated fever	Yes	Yes	Possible	No	No
Low oxygen saturation	Possible	Yes	Yes	Possible	No

Recommended Investigations

** FBC: leukocytosis suggests bacterial infection, common in asthma; eosinophilia in allergy

** Sputum for culture from children with productive cough

** Lung function testing, spirometry and peak flow measurements

** Chest X-ray is very helpful in diagnosing pneumonia, foreign body

** CT scan of the lung to diagnose bronchiectasis

** Sweat test if CF is suspected

** Bronchoscopy for unexplained cough

** Gastric pH study for cases suspected of having GO reflux

Top Tips

- Cough is usually self-limited and the focus should be directed at the cause of the cough, not at the symptom cough. Educate parents that 'cough medicines' are unlikely to help children with cough.
- Children's cough is rarely productive, therefore the term *wet cough* rather than *productive cough* is more appropriate.
- Although wheezing with cough is usually present in asthma, cough may be the only symptom, which characteristically worsens with activity and at night.
- If the cough is persistent and a diagnosis has not been established, a trial with a bronchodilator is worthwhile; sometimes inhaled steroid is helpful.
- Protracted bacterial bronchitis (PBB) is commonly found in young children with chronic cough that worsens when changing posture. There is no abnormality on physical examination or on chest X-ray. The condition improves on antibiotics for 2 weeks.
- In a child with pertussis-like cough, who is fully immunised, adenovirus and other viruses may have caused the illness. The classical 'whoop' is often not present in immunised children.
- Children with bronchiectasis present with chronic wet cough, recurrent chest infections and often with intermittent purulent sputum and haemoptysis. Finger clubbing and crackles on chest auscultation are often found.
- All children with chronic cough should have lung function tests, chest X-ray and oxygen saturation performed.
- A psychogenic or habit cough is typically loud and repetitive (often seen as throat clearing), absent during sleep and unresponsive to any medication. Duration may be a few weeks or months.

Red Flags

- The possibility of foreign body always has to be considered with chronic and unexplained cough in young children. If missed, bronchiectasis is likely to ensue.
- A child who presents with cough on exertion only could have asthma. Peak flow measurements before and after exercise, with and without a bronchodilator, will help establish the diagnosis.
- A severe coughing paroxysm causing high intrathoracic pressure and reduced venous return, manifesting as a red face, may result in cerebral hypoxia and syncope.
- Cases of protracted bacterial bronchitis are often misdiagnosed as asthma, resulting in a persistence of symptoms that can lead to bronchiectasis.
- An underweight child with chronic cough should undergo sweat test to exclude CF.
- Children with developmental delay may present with persistent cough due to aspiration and aspiration pneumonia. The cough can mimic and be misdiagnosed as asthma or bronchitis.

FURTHER READING

Weinberger M, Lockshin B. When is cough functional, and how should be treated. *Breathe (Sheff)* 2017;13(1):22–30.

COUGHING UP BLOOD (HAEMOPTYSIS)

Clinical Overview

Haemoptysis is defined as coughing or expectoration of blood or the presence of blood-tinged sputum. It is always a frightening experience for patients and their parents, warranting immediate diagnostic attention. In contrast to adults, haemoptysis is not a common symptom in children and is usually not life threatening. There are numerous causes of haemoptysis, which usually can be diagnosed by obtaining a careful history, physical examination and laboratory testing. In general, the source of the bleeding is from either the lungs or the bronchial system. The amount of bleeding from the lung tends to be small compared to the bleeding from the bronchi, which produce a larger quantity of blood. Extrapulmonary causes of haemoptysis are rare but may include nasopharyngeal infection or foreign body in the upper airways. Haemoptysis must be differentiated from epistaxis and haematemesis.

Possible Diagnoses

Infants	Children
Common	
Side effect of surfactant pulmonary	Pneumonia
Post-intubation	Coagulopathy
Disseminated intravascular coagulopathy	CF
Coagulopathy	Vigorous cough
Pulmonary oedema	Foreign body (FB) (mostly <4 years of age)
Rare	
	Bronchiectasis
	Pulmonary embolism
	Pulmonary oedema
	Lung abscess
	Pulmonary tuberculosis
	Left ventricular heart failure (mitral stenosis)
	Goodpasture's syndrome
	Wegener's granulomatosis
	Hereditary haemorrhagic telangiectasia
	Pulmonary vascular malformation
	Hydatid cyst
	Pulmonary tumours (adenoma, haemartoma)
	Sarcoidosis
	Connective tissue diseases (particularly systemic lupus erythematosus [SLE])
	Haemosiderosis
	Mycetoma

Differential Diagnosis at a Glance

	Pneumonia	Coagulopathy	CF	Vigorous Cough	FB
Massive bleeding	No	Possible	No	No	Possible
Short history	Yes	Possible	No	Yes	Yes
Associated fever	Yes	No	Possible	Possible	Possible
Bleeding elsewhere	No	Yes	No	No	No
Previous haemoptysis	No	Yes	Possible	No	No

Recommended Investigations

** FBC: low Hb to confirm anaemia; leukocytosis in pneumonia; low platelet in thrombocytopenia

*** Coagulation study with international normalised ratio, prothrombin time and partial thromboplastin time in case of coagulopathy

** Auto-antibody screen may be positive for connective tissue diseases

** Sputum cytology for suspected Tb or tumour

*** Chest X-ray (the most valuable investigation) to find the cause of the haemoptysis

*** Sweat test for suspected cases of CF

** Bronchoscopy and high-resolution CT scan of the lungs in unclear cases of haemoptysis

Top Tips

• Haemoptysis in young children is usually caused by benign conditions such as vigorous cough.
• After a careful history and physical examination, a chest X-ray should be performed. If the diagnosis is not clear: bronchoscopy and chest CT scan and referral to a chest specialist.
• A child with haemoptysis and high fever is most likely having pneumonia.
• The low-pressure pulmonary system tends to produce a non-profuse haemoptysis while the bronchi, which are at systemic pressure, tend to produce more massive bleeding.
• Haemoptysis (with history of lung disease, frothy, bright-red, absence of nausea and vomiting) should be easily differentiated from haematemesis (with history of gastric or hepatic disease, coffee-ground, brown to red, presence of nausea and vomiting, mixed with food particles).
• About 5% of patients with CF may develop haemoptysis, which may recur.
• Tuberculosis is on the increase in the United Kingdom; the disease should not be forgotten as a cause of haemoptysis.

Red Flags

• When a child presents with haemoptysis, look for clubbing of the fingers to identify CF.
• Young children under 5 years swallow their sputum and the minor haemoptysis may not be obvious, unless the haemoptysis is massive.
• Beware that among obscure causes of haemoptysis is left-ventricular heart failure or mitral stenosis causing pulmonary hypertension.
• Pulmonary embolism may cause haemoptysis. Consider this diagnosis if there is evidence of deep vein thrombosis or the child is at risk of thrombosis, such as SCA or homocystinuria.
• Factitious haemoptysis is rare but should be considered in the differential diagnosis of unclear cause of haemoptysis when the medical history or the patient's behaviour is unusual.

FURTHER READING

Sim J, Kim H, Lee H et al. Etiology of hemoptysis in children: A single institutional series of 40 cases. *Allergy Asthma Immunol Res* 2009;1(1):41–44.

NIPPLE DISCHARGE

Clinical Overview

Unless the cause of nipple discharge is obvious (e.g. local inflammation or medication induced), this phenomenon must be carefully evaluated, as for adults. Although the condition is usually alarming for parents, fortunately its causes are usually benign in children. Discharge may be persistent or intermittent, scant or abundant, free flowing or elicited by nipple stimulation, and unilateral or bilateral. It is due to a variety of causes. In general, milky discharge, thick or not, suggests a benign condition (except galactorrhoea due to pituitary prolactinoma), while purulent discharge suggests infection, and serous or bloody discharge may suggest mastitis, mammary duct ectasia, intraductal papilloma or rarely cancer. Duct ectasia is the most common cause of bloody discharge.

Possible Diagnoses

Infants	Children
Common	
Physiological	Local stimulation
Mastitis	Mammary duct ectasia
Areola abscess	Medications (e.g. contraceptives)
Medication induced	Breast infection (mastitis, abscess)
Mammary duct ectasia	Galactorrhoea
Rare	
	Pregnancy
	Breast cancer (adenocarcinoma)
	Prolactin-secreting pituitary tumour
	Intraductal papilloma
	Fibroadenoma
	Hypothyroidism
	Fibrocystic breast disease
	Injury to the breast
	Idiopathic

Differential Diagnosis at a Glance

	Local Stimulation	Mammary Duct Ectasia	Drugs	Breast Infection	Galactorrhoea
Common in adolescents	Yes	Possible	Possible	Possible	Possible
Bilateral	Possible	No	Yes	No	Possible
Occur in boys	Possible	Possible	Yes	Possible	Possible
CNS symptoms (e.g. headache)	No	No	No	No	No
Bloody discharge	Possible	Yes	No	Yes	No

Recommended Investigations

*** Prolactin level to check for hyperprolactinaemia; thyroid function test (TFT) to check for hypothyroidism

*** Microscopic examination to confirm galactorrhoea by finding the presence of fat globules; culture of the discharge is indicated for purulent discharge
*** Pregnancy test to be considered for post-puberty girls if clinically indicated
*** Ultrasound scan is the best imaging investigation and is an essential diagnostic tool
*** Cranial MRI to exclude hyperprolactinaemia

Top Tips

- The presence of more than two breasts, termed *polymastia* (or supernumerary), is found in up to 6% of the population. It is seen along the embryological milk lines, which extend from the axilla to the inguinal region, leaving later two segments that become breasts. Failure to regress causes ectopic or supernumerary breast tissue.
- Galactorrhoea is a discharge of milk or milk-like secretion from the breast, unrelated to childbirth or nursing. In the neonates, nipple discharge (witch's milk) should be regarded as physiological and is best left alone, as manipulation may cause mastitis.
- Idiopathic galactorrhoea is a diagnosis of exclusion and should not be diagnosed easily unless other possible underlying conditions have been eliminated by thorough history, examination and laboratory evaluation.
- Benign conditions of the breast with nipple discharge include abnormal response of the breast tissue to maternal hormones and intraductal papilloma. Mammary duct ectasia is the most common cause of bloody nipple discharge in the paediatric population.
- Examination of the discharge assists in diagnosis: in benign conditions it is usually milky thick or clear; infection is associated with purulent discharge; and in cancer it is usually serous or bloody.
- History of any medication should be obtained. Medications which may cause galactorrhoea include metoclopramide, tricyclic antidepressants, phenothiazines or contraceptive pills.

Red Flags

- In galactorrhoea (spontaneous flow of milk), pituitary prolactinoma may be the underlying pathology, which is among the most common type of pituitary tumours. CNS examination should be performed, including visual examination, to exclude tumours. Prolactin level correlates well with the tumour size; a serum prolactin level >200 ng/mL is abnormal.
- Swelling in the axilla, chest wall or even in the vulva may be due to supernumerary breasts. Although they are benign, distinction from other benign or malignant masses is necessary.
- Bloody nipple discharge may suggest inflammatory breast conditions (mastitis), duct ectasia and intraductal papilloma. These may mimic breast cancer and should be considered.
- Duct ectasia may resolve spontaneously within 3–9 months. Any surgical intervention should be considered very carefully because of the damage to the normal developing bud tissue.
- Hypothyroidism is second after pituitary pathology in causing galactorrhoea. Thyroid function tests should be carried out for any obscure case of nipple discharge.

FURTHER READING

Nascimento M, Portela A, Espada F et al. Bloody nipple discharge in infancy – A report of two cases. *BMJ Case Rep* 2012;2012:bcr2012006649.
Singal R, Mehta SK, Bala J et al. A study of evaluation and management of rare congenital breast diseases. *J Clin Diagn Res* 2016;10(10):PC18–PC24.

PALPITATION

Clinical Overview

Cardiologists may use the term *palpitation* to describe an awareness of the heartbeat due to abnormality of the heart rhythm ranging from simple, benign ectopic atrial or ventricular beats to more important tachyarrhythmias and life-threatening cardiac diseases. Patients may use the term to describe a perception or awareness of irregular, fast or skipped heartbeats, or simple awareness of their pulse, particularly when it is fast or when lying on one side in bed. A young child who cannot explain the event by words may stop his or her normal activity, expressing discomfort or clinching the left side of the chest. Palpitation is usually a terrifying experience for children and for their parents. In paediatric practise, the differential diagnosis is usually narrowed between tachycardia (such as SVT), ectopic beats and cardiac diseases. Any palpitation with a history of syncope without warning is most likely of cardiac origin (ventricular tachycardia). In such case, an urgent evaluation is essential.

Possible Diagnoses

Infants	Children
Common	
Sinus arrhythmia	Sinus tachycardia (fever, exercise)
Premature atrial contractions	Anxiety
	Anaemia
	Arrhythmia (such as ectopic beats, SVT)
	Drugs (e.g. bronchodilators, use of stimulants)
Rare	
SVT	Thyrotoxicosis
Ventricular tachycardia	Heart diseases (cardiomyopathy)
Neonatal Graves' disease	Electrolytes disturbance
	Pheochromocytoma
	Carcinoid syndrome
	Hypoglycaemia (e.g. from insulinoma)

Differential Diagnosis at a Glance

	Sinus Tachycardia	Anxiety	Anaemia	Arrhythmia	Drugs
Short (few minutes) episode	No	Possible	No	Possible	No
Regular rhythm	Yes	Yes	Yes	No	Yes
Associated pallor	No	Possible	Yes	Possible	No
Diagnosis requires ECG	No	No	Yes	Yes	Possible
Associated tremor	No	Possible	No	No	Yes

Recommended Investigations

*** ECG to diagnose arrhythmia, e.g. SVT, sinus tachycardia or Wolff–Parkinson–White (WPW) syndrome; 24-hour ECG
*** FBC to check the Hb for anaemia
*** TFTs to diagnose hyperthyroidism

** Urea and electrolytes (U&E) mainly to check for a potassium level that may aggravate arrhythmia

** A chest X-ray may be helpful showing cardiac enlargement in case of failure

** Treadmill exercise test may help reveal any exercise-induced arrhythmia

Top Tips

- Sinus arrhythmia (increasing heartbeats in inspiration, slowing down in expiration) is normal in neonates and older children; it becomes accentuated during activities.
- If the history suggests arrhythmia and examination is normal, 24-hour ECG monitor is indicated.
- Most patients with palpitation do not have a cardiac lesion.
- Although a diagnosis of cardiac arrhythmia can often be made during the attack, between attacks heart and ECG may be entirely normal. Exceptions to this are WPW syndrome, associated with SVT, and long QT syndrome.
- The treatment of attention deficit hyperactivity disorder with stimulants (methylphenidate, amphetamine) has been a common practise for decades. Common side effects include insomnia, nervousness and palpitation.
- In considering the differential diagnosis of palpitation due to arrhythmia, the two important common diagnoses are SVT or ectopic beats. Ectopic beats are harmless, provided there is no heart disease, anaemia or thyrotoxicosis. Sudden onset of tachycardia in association with dizziness and dyspnoea is very suggestive of SVT.
- It is uncertain whether sport participation is a risk factor for sudden cardiac death (SCD), as SCD may also occur in recreational activity, quiet time and sleep.

Red Flags

- The normal pulse of an awake infant younger than 3 months ranges between 100 and 220/minute. Sinus arrhythmia is normal, and it is abnormal for a child not to have sinus arrhythmia.
- A child with palpitation and pallor with a heart murmur should not be diagnosed as having cardiac disease; the murmur may be a haemic functional murmur, which disappears once the anaemia is corrected.
- Palpitation is more serious if it is associated with chest pain, shortness of breath, fainting or in the presence of cardiac disease. Urgent evaluation is needed.
- SVT in a young child presents as CCF. Conversion SVT to sinus rhythm is urgently required.
- Beware that palpitation could occasionally be a risk factor for sudden cardiac death in the young. Other associated features include episodes of chest pain, syncope and long QT syndrome in the ECG.
- Pheochromocytoma is rare but potentially fatal unless recognised and treated. Children may present with sweating, syncope and palpitation.

FURTHER READING

Ackerman M, Atkins DL, Triedman JK. Sudden cardiac death in the young. *Circulation* 2016;133(10): 1006–1026.

RESPIRATORY NOISES

Clinical Overview

Although respiratory noises as reported by the parents are extremely common, these noises are often difficult to be differentiated from each other. The difficulty is compounded by the fact that children may have multiple noises, being intermittent and changing from one noise to another in a few minutes or according to awake or sleep position (polyphonic). Clinicians should realise that it is very common that when parents report a type of noise, e.g. wheezing, it is often not confirmed. It is important to know that snuffles and stridor are caused by obstruction of the extrathoracic airways (nose, pharynx, larynx and the extrathoracic portion of the trachea), while wheezing is caused by intrathoracic obstruction. Clinicians should be familiar with a few common noises (wheeze, stridor, rattle, grunt, snore and snuffle) and must be confident when diagnosing these specific types of noises. An error in recognising specific types of noises will lead to diagnostic and therapeutic errors.

Possible Diagnoses

Infants	Children
Common	
Snuffles	Wheeze
Stridor	Stridor
Grunt	Rattle
Wheeze	Snore
Rattle	Grunt
Rare	
Mew	Snuffle
	Purr
	Moan
	Squeak

Differential Diagnosis at a Glance

	Wheeze	Stridor	Grunt	Rattle	Snore
Ill looking	Possible	Possible	Yes	No	No
Expiratory	Yes	No	Yes	Yes	No
Inspiratory	Possible	Yes	No	Yes	Yes
Associated cough	Yes	Possible	Possible	Possible	No
Worse at night	Yes	Yes	Possible	Possible	Yes

Recommended Investigations

** FBC: leukocytosis, and blood culture if the stridor is suspected to be due to epiglottitis

*** Blood for chromosomal analysis if cri-du-chat is suspected

** Chest X-ray often required with more persistent symptoms

*** Lung function tests: in persistent wheezing; peak flow measurement in children older than 5 years

** Direct laryngoscopy for unusual features of stridor

** Video recording the respiratory noises by the parents is helpful to differentiate noises

Top Tips

- Acute snuffles are mostly due to a viral infection, while persistent ones are due to allergic rhinitis, adenoid hypertrophy or snuffles of infancy. The latter noise is so common that it can be regarded as 'normal'; it has no discharge and usually disappears between ages 3 and 6 months.
- When parents report their child has a wheeze, the clinician must confirm it. Children may have rattles or stridor. Doctors should imitate a wheeze, or to ask the parents to imitate the sound.
- Extrathoracic obstruction produces inspiratory stridor while the intrathoracic obstruction produces wheeze. The association of hoarseness and stridor suggests an obstruction at the vocal cords of the larynx; when cough is present, the trachea is involved.
- Laryngomalacia is the most common cause of chronic stridor, noted usually soon after birth, and disappears at the age of 12–18 months. It is not associated with cough, failure to thrive or feeding problems. It does not need a laryngoscopy to confirm it unless there are atypical features.
- Hoarseness in laryngomalacia is not present because vocal cords are not involved. Hoarseness with stridor is very suggestive of laryngotracheobronchitis.
- A rare syndrome that produces high-pitched mewing cry, closely resembling the cry of a kitten, is cri-du-chat, due to a deletion of the short arm of chromosome 5.
- A rattle noise should not be considered an asthma symptom: if acute it is due to viral infection; if persistent it is due to GO reflux, or sputum retention found in neuromuscular diseases.

Red Flags

- Persistent snuffles are often misdiagnosed as cold, and many topical medications, such as sprays, are prescribed unnecessarily, and some are harmful.
- Persistent nasal snuffles need to be differentiated from partial choanal atresia. In older children, polyps need to be excluded. If a polyp is found, CF has to be ruled out.
- The term *snuffles* was first used for children with congenital syphilis. Although this infection is rare, it is on the rise, and it may present with the triad of anaemia, snuffle and splenomegaly.
- A diagnosis of inhalation of a foreign body causing stridor or wheezing should never be missed.
- A major error is misdiagnosing stridor from an upper airway obstruction as wheeze, leading to incorrect treatment that can be life threatening.
- In contrast to other respiratory noises, expiratory grunt is usually a serous sign seen in neonates in association with respiratory distress syndrome, and in older children with pneumonia.

FURTHER READING

Maguire A, Gopalabaje S, Eastham K. All that wheezes is not asthma: A 6-year-old with foreign body aspiration and no suggestive history. *BMJ Case Rep* 2012;2012:bcr2012006640.

2 ABDOMEN

ACUTE ABDOMINAL PAIN

Clinical Overview

Acute abdominal pain is one of the most common symptoms in children. The main objective in dealing with acute abdominal pain is to differentiate between benign self-limited conditions, such as constipation or gastroenteritis, and more life-threatening surgical conditions such as volvulus or appendicitis. The term *acute abdomen* refers to an intra-abdominal condition, which usually requires a surgical intervention, such as appendicitis. This accounts for around 1% of all children presenting with acute abdominal pain. Pain is classified as visceral pain that is usually dull, poorly localized and perceived in the midline in response to mechanical (stretching or ischaemia) and chemical stimuli. Visceral pain originating from the foregut (e.g. lower oesophagus, stomach) is typically felt in the epigastric area; pain originating from the midgut (e.g. small intestine) is typically felt in the peri-umbilical area; and pain originating from the hindgut (e.g. colon) is typically felt in the lower abdomen. Somatic pain receptors are located in the parietal peritoneum, muscle and skin, which transmit pain via the spinal cord from T6 to L1. Somatic pain is typically sharp, intense and well localised. Referred pain is felt in distant areas of the same cutaneous dermatome as the affected organs, e.g. pneumonia or pharyngitis causing abdominal pain. Pain can be sharp and localised or a vague ache.

Possible Diagnoses

Infants	Children
Common	
Hunger	GE
Infection elsewhere (ear)	Psychogenic (e.g. anxiety, school phobia)
Urinary tract infection (UTI)	Constipation
Gastroenteritis (GE)	Appendicitis
Evening colic	Mesenteric adenitis (MA)
	Migraine
Rare	
Incarcerated hernia	Referred pain (e.g. pneumonia, pharyngitis)
Intussusception	UTI
Intestinal obstruction	Renal stones
Meckel's diverticulum	Pancreatitis
Volvulus	Trauma
Trauma	Testicular/ovarian torsion
Inborn error of metabolism	Peritonitis
Imperforate hymen	Incarcerated hernia
	Meckel's diverticulum
	Henoch–Schönlein's purpura (HSP)

(Continued)

(Continued)

Infants	Children
	Hepatitis
	Intussusception
	Intestinal obstruction
	Crohn's disease (CD)
	Diabetic ketoacidosis (DKA)
	Sickle cell anaemia
	Gall bladder stones

Differential Diagnosis at a Glance

	GE	Psychogenic	Constipation	Appendicitis	Mesenteric Adenitis
Diarrhoea	Yes	No	No	Possible	No
Diffuse pain	Yes	Yes	Yes	No	No
Abdominal tenderness	Possible	Possible	Possible	Yes	Yes
Localised pain	No	No	No	Yes	No
Fever	Possible	No	No	Yes	Yes

Recommended Investigations

*** Urinalysis and culture to confirm UTI
*** Stool culture for bacterial GE; viral antigen detection for rotavirus
**   Full blood count (FBC): leukocytosis suggests inflammatory or infectious causes
*** Serum amylase/lipase for suspected pancreatitis
*** Liver function tests to diagnose hepatitis, blood glucose, urea and electrolytes (U&E) and blood gases for DKA
**   Abdominal plain X-ray confirms impacted stool masses in constipation, signs of bowel obstruction
*** Abdominal ultrasound for suspected renal or gall bladder stones
*** Barium enema or air-contrast enema for cases with suspected intussusception

Top Tips

- Abdominal examination should be performed with extreme gentleness and compassion; careful hands-off inspection being the first step, followed by non-intimidating position of sitting down or kneeling to be at the same level with the child. A young child is best examined in a parent's arms or lap. Distracting the child while palpating the abdomen is very helpful.
- A student or postgraduate doctor in an examination who hurts the child while examining the abdomen should expect to fail.
- It is worth asking the child to point with his/her finger to the area 'where it hurts most'.
- The closer the pain to the umbilicus, the less likely it is to be organic disease.
- The use of sedative or analgesic does not increase the risk of misdiagnosis.
- Urinalysis is essential in a febrile child with acute abdominal pain, particularly if the fever has no localised source.
- Children with appendicitis present initially with vague abdominal pain, poorly localised in the peri-umbilical area, followed by nausea. Within 6–48 hours, the pain migrates to the right lower quadrant followed by vomiting and fever.
- Typical abdomen in GE is non-distended, soft and mildly tender, with mid-abdominal cramping but little or no guarding. Vomiting usually precedes the diarrhoea by as much as 12–24 hours.

- In cases of mesenteric adenitis, stool culture for the bacteria *Yersinia* should be performed.
- Meckel's diverticulum affects 2% of the population, and of these 2% become symptomatic. About 60% of diverticula contain heterotopic gastric or endometrial tissue that can cause symptoms.

Red Flags

- The clinician's skills must be used to differentiate between a self-limited process (e.g. viral gastroenteritis, constipation) and more life-threatening surgical emergencies (e.g. intussusception). Overlooking a serious organic aetiology is a major concern.
- Bilious vomiting must always be taken seriously because of possible malrotation or volvulus.
- Extra-abdominal conditions (e.g. tonsillitis, lower lobe pneumonia, testicular disease, spine or hip synovitis) can produce abdominal pain mimicking abdominal emergencies, e.g. appendicitis. Examination of these sites is essential.
- Be aware that a young child with appendicitis may present with diarrhoea only.
- Children with MA may present with acute abdominal pain in the lower quadrant of the abdomen mimicking appendicitis, but pain is more diffuse in MA. If in doubt, appendectomy should be considered.
- Because of difficulty in evaluating the abdomen in young children with appendicitis, they often present with acute abdomen due to perforation. Perforation rates are high in this age group. Children typically have a longer history of pain, greater systemic effect, high fever, more generalized tenderness and absent bowel sounds.
- A young child with mild abdominal pain and vomiting who has clinical signs of dehydration but no ketones in the urine should be investigated to rule out an inborn error of metabolism.

FURTHER READING

Yang WC, Chen CY, Wu HP. Etiology of non-traumatic acute abdomen in pediatric emergency departments. *World J Clin Cases* 2013;1(9):276–284.

RECURRENT ABDOMINAL PAIN

Clinical Overview

Recurrent abdominal pain (RAP) is a common symptom affecting 10%–20% of children; school-age children (5–14 years) have the highest incidence. Recently (Rome criteria), the term of *functional gastrointestinal disorders* (FGIDs) was introduced and includes irritable bowel syndrome (constipation predominately, diarrhoea predominately or mixed); functional dyspepsia (epigastric pain, postprandial distress, early satiation); abdominal migraine (peri-umbilical pain lasting at least an hour, with pallor, nausea, vomiting, anorexia and headache); and functional abdominal pain. RAP is significant because it causes a high rate of morbidity, missed school days, high use of health resources and parental anxiety. It was defined as 'at least 3 recurrent episodes of pain, severe enough to affect child's activities, over a period of at least 3 months, and the symptoms cannot be attributed to another medical condition' (Apley's criteria); Apley in 1958 estimated that only 8% of patients had RAP. Nowadays, a higher estimate is accepted mainly because irritable bowel syndrome (IBS) has been recognised as an important cause of RAP, and because of a high rate of detecting pathology by newer imaging technology. Parasites, such as *Giardia*, are a common and important cause of RAP in developing countries. Most children with RAP have no organic diseases (functional abdominal pain). Non-organic causes are typically central to the abdomen, with no guarding, rebound, rigidity or abnormal physical signs or investigation. Recurrent crying episodes in an infant who draws the legs up and appears to be in pain are defined as colic.

Possible Diagnoses

Infants	Children
Common	
Infantile colic (evening colic)	Functional (psychogenic, e.g. school phobia)
Gastro-oesophageal (GO) reflux	IBS
Lactose intolerance	Food intolerance/allergy
Cow's milk protein allergy	Abdominal migraine (cyclic vomiting syndrome)
Parasites (*Giardia*)	Parasites (*Giardia*)
Rare	
Coeliac disease	Inflammatory bowel diseases (IBDs) (CD, ulcerative colitis)
Meckel's diverticulum	Recurrent urinary tract infection
Child abuse	Familial Mediterranean fever
Scurvy	Child abuse
Sickle cell anaemia (SCA)	Porphyria
	SCA
	Coeliac disease
	Meckel's diverticulum
	Pancreatitis
	Choledochal cyst
	Hepatitis
	Stones in the urinary system and gall bladder
	Lead poisoning
	Peptic ulcer
	Wilms' tumour

Differential Diagnosis at a Glance

	Functional RAP	IBS	Food Intolerance	Abdominal Migraine	Parasites (*Giardia*)
Weight loss	No	No	Possible	No	Possible
Bloody diarrhoea	No	No	Possible	No	Possible
Stool changes	No	Yes	Yes	No	Possible
Vomiting	No	No	Possible	Yes	Possible
Cause of malabsorption	No	No	Possible	No	Yes

Recommended Investigations

*** Urinalysis: haematuria suggests renal stones; leukocytes and nitrite suggest UTI

** Stool for parasites and culture; screening testing for *Helicobacter pylori*

** Stool calprotectin to differentiate between IBD and IBS

** FBC with C-reactive protein (CRP): useful in suggesting inflammation and infection; anaemia in SCA

** Liver function tests (to diagnose hepatitis, Gilbert's syndrome); coeliac screening tests

*** Abdominal ultrasound scan to confirm renal or gall bladder stones, and tumours

Top Tips

- The closer the pain is to the umbilicus, the less likely it is to be significant. Pain away from the umbilicus is suggestive of organic causes.
- Children of parents with gastrointestinal (GI) disease, children with stress and children with obesity or previous abdominal surgery are more likely to have RAP.
- Functional abdominal diseases are suggested by a symptom-free interval, the healthy appearance of the child and an absence of abnormalities on examination. Organic diseases tend to have a progressive course and the presence of abnormalities on examination.
- Pain that is followed, not preceded, by vomiting is suggestive of appendicitis.
- Infant colic is defined as irritability paroxysms with fussiness or crying that starts and ends without clear reasons, lasting at least 3 h/day, 3 days/week, for at least 3 weeks in a healthy baby.
- IBS accounts for the majority of paediatric RAP, and is due to dysregulation of visceral neural pathways, leading to visceral hyperalgesia. Infection or stress may trigger this sensitisation.
- Clinical presentation of IBD often overlaps with IBS. Stool calprotectin has proved to be very useful in the differential diagnosis between IBD and IBS: low calprotectin makes IBD unlikely.
- Pain in constipation is often overrated as a diagnostic entity. It should not be considered simply because no other cause except constipation is elicited from the history and examination.
- Note that food intolerance/allergy is among the most common causes of RAP in an otherwise healthy child. Eliminating the suspected food item (particularly milk or wheat) for about 2 weeks is the best diagnostic and therapeutic tool. Blood or skin testing is of limited value.
- Psychogenic causes should be diagnosed on positive grounds, not by excluding organic disease. Parents should not hear 'the cause is psychological'. They should be supported by being offered reassurance that their child is healthy and the abdominal pain will not affect his/her well-being.

Red Flags

- A child known to have recurrent functional abdominal pain could present one day with an organic cause which may need surgical intervention.
- Alarm features that suggest organic causes include children younger than 4 years of age, weight loss, falling off growth centile, persistent pain in the right or left upper or right lower quadrant of the abdomen or in the supra-pubic area, or association with vomiting, persistent diarrhoea or fever.
- Other alarm features include a family history of inflammatory bowel diseases, pain associated with dysphagia or heartburn or with night-waking, oral and/or perianal lesions or arthritis that suggest non-functional causes of abdominal pain.
- Remember that the frequency of RAP and the duration of symptoms are often longer in children who were victims of sexual abuse. If such a case is suspected, the child should be protected in a hospital environment until the diagnosis is conclusively made.

FURTHER READING

Horst S, Shelby G, Anderson J et al. Predicting persistence of functional abdominal pain from childhood into young adulthood. *Clin Gastroenterol Hepatol* 2014;12(12):2026–2032.
Korterink JJ, Diederson K, Benninga MA et al. Epidemiology of pediatric functional abdominal pain disorders: A meta-analysis. *PLOS ONE* 2015;10(5):e0126982.

ABDOMINAL DISTENSION

Clinical Overview

Abdominal distension is defined as an increase of girth of the abdomen caused by air, fluid, stool, mass or organomegaly. It is a common clinical finding that must be evaluated carefully. History is of paramount importance in giving a diagnostic clue, e.g. duration of the distension (acute or chronic?), any weight loss, diarrhoea or vomiting (and is the vomiting bile stained?). Many toddlers, who are thriving and well, often have a mild and harmless abdominal distension. This condition may be associated with toddler's diarrhoea. A long history of abdominal distension associated with underweight and loose motions is very suggestive of malabsorption, and coeliac disease is the most common cause. Vomiting, particularly bile stained, suggests intestinal obstruction.

Possible Diagnoses

Infants	Children
Common	
Mechanical ventilation	Physiological in toddlers (usually mild)
Necrotising enterocolitis (NEC)	Malabsorption (coeliac disease, *Giardia*)
Intestinal atresia or stenosis	Intestinal obstruction
Meconium plug or ileus	Constipation
Abdominal mass (tumour, hepatosplenomegaly)	Abdominal mass (e.g. hepatic or renal)
Rare	
Sepsis	Glycogen storage disease
Hepatomegaly, splenomegaly	Hirschsprung's disease
Tumour (nephroblastoma, neuroblastoma)	Ascites (e.g. nephrotic syndrome, systemic lupus erythematosus)
Imperforate hymen	Ovarian cyst
Hydrometrocolpos	Kwashiorkor
Gartner's duct cyst	Hydatid cyst
Prolapsed ureterocele, urethrocele	Aerophagia (functional or pathological)
Chloramphenicol toxicity (gray syndrome)	Postoperative abdominal distension
Renal vein thrombosis (flank mass)	Abdominal (peritoneal) tuberculosis
	Cystic fibrosis (CF)
	Polycystic renal disease

Differential Diagnosis at a Glance

	Physiological (in toddlers)	Malabsorption	Intestinal Obstruction	Constipation	Abdominal Mass
Thriving	Yes	No	Yes	Yes	Possible
Diarrhoea	No	Yes	No	No	No
Palpable mass	No	No	Possible	Yes	Yes
Failure to thrive	No	Yes	No	No	No
Vomiting	Possible	Yes	Yes	Yes	Possible

Recommended Investigations

*** Stool microscopy for *Giardia*, pus cells and stool culture
**   FBC, CRP to screen for infection; blood culture to rule out sepsis, screening tests for CD

**   Abdominal X-ray for constipation and intestinal obstruction, and for detection of tumor
***   Ultrasound scan to confirm abdominal masses, e.g. renal mass, ovarian cyst
**   Barium enema may suggest Hirschsprung's disease; rectal biopsy confirms it
***   Computed tomography or magnetic resonance imaging to evaluate abdominal masses, ascites, organomegaly
**   Sweat test for cystic fibrosis

Top Tips

- In functional gut disorders: abdominal distension is often associated with bloating (about 50%). Bloating is a subjective sensation of increased abdominal pressure without an increase in abdominal girth; distension is associated with similar sensation but with increased girth.
- Although hydronephrosis and multicystic dysplastic kidney are the two most common abdominal masses, they do not cause abdominal distension.
- Be aware of two important causes of chronic distension: malabsorption and coeliac disease.
- Causes of abdominal distension in the tropics differ from those in developed countries; there parasites (e.g. *Giardia*, hydatid cyst) and kwashiorkor may prevail.
- A lower intestinal obstruction (e.g. Hirschsprung's disease) usually presents with abdominal distension and late vomiting, while an upper one presents with early vomiting and no distension.
- Functional aerophagia refers to excessive air swallowing without significant GI symptoms, whereas pathological aerophagia is associated with abdominal pain, belching, burping and flatulence. Typical presentation in both conditions: no abdominal distension in the morning, followed by progressive abdominal distension during the day.

Red Flags

- Excluding toddler's physiologic abdominal distension and aerophagia, abdominal distension should always be considered serious, requiring usually urgent investigations.
- The priority remains to exclude life-threatening surgical causes of abdominal distension such as intestinal obstruction.
- A child who has failed to thrive with abdominal distension should not be considered physiologic; the most likely cause is malabsorption.
- Bilious vomiting must be taken seriously because of the possibility of malrotation with volvulus.

FURTHER READING

Morabito G, Romeo C, Romano C. Functional aerophagia in children: A frequent, atypical disorder. *Case Rep Gastroenterol* 2014;8(1):123–128.

CONSTIPATION

Clinical Overview

Constipation is a term used to describe infrequent (two or fewer) defecations per week or hard stools which are difficult to pass. It is often associated with a history of retentive posturing, painful defecation, large-diameter stools and large faecal mass in the rectum. It is important to remember that infrequent defecation is common in breast-fed babies who may not have a stool for 10 days. There should be no intervention as long as babies are thriving, feeding well, have no abdominal distension and pass stools without pain or blood. In older children, the most common reason is withholding stool for fear of having a bowel movement following an experience of a painful defecation. A diet insufficient in fiber intake and poor toilet training play a role. Faecal incontinence is a common complication (about 80%) and is defined as voluntary or involuntary passage of faeces into the underwear or in socially inappropriate places, in a child with a developmental age of at least 4 years. Faecal incontinence not related to constipation (non-retentive) and organic causes (e.g. anorectal malformation) is comparatively uncommon.

Differential Diagnosis

Infants	Children
Common	
Normal variant in breast-fed	Chronic habitual constipation
Insufficient fluid intake, dehydration	Prolonged febrile illness
Neurodisability (CP, myotonica dystrophica)	Increased output (e.g. polyuria, vomiting)
Intestinal obstruction (e.g. meconium ileus, plug)	Neurodisability (CP, myotonica dystrophica)
Change from breast to bottle feeding	IBS
Persistent vomiting (e.g. pyloric stenosis)	
Rare	
Hirschsprung's disease	Polyuria
Hypothyroidism	Recurrent or chronic vomiting
Hypercalcaemia	Hypercalcaemia
Intestinal stricture	Hirschsprung's disease (HD)
Anteriorly displaced anus	Drugs, such as narcotics, antidepressant
Imperforate anus	Prader-Willi syndrome
Any cause of polyuria (renal tubular acidosis)	Coeliac disease

Differential Diagnosis at a Glance

	Functional Constipation	Prolonged Febrile Illness	Increased Loss (e.g. vomiting)	Neurodisability	IBS
Only symptom	Possible	No	No	No	Possible
With faecal incontinence	Yes	No	No	Possible	No
Mild symptom	Possible	Yes	Possible	Possible	Yes
Associated loose stools	Possible (overflow)	No	No	Possible	Yes
Short history	Possible	No	Possible	No	No

Recommended Investigations

** Urinalysis to exclude an associated UTI
** Plain abdominal X-ray: may show distended bowel and rectum (megacolon) full of faeces
** Thyroid function text and serum calcium to exclude hypothyroidism and hypercalcaemia
** Rectal biopsy if there is clinical suspicion of Hirschsprung's disease

Top Tips

- By far the most common cause of constipation is functional; organic diseases (Hirschsprung's disease, hypothyroidism, hypercalcaemia, renal tubular acidosis) are rare in practice (<5%).
- Looking at the child can give important clues to the underlying diagnosis (e.g. hypothyroidism, failure to thrive, distended abdomen in Hirschsprung's disease, or elfin face in hypercalcaemia).
- Parents often interpret withholding stool as pushing; explanation should be given for that.
- Although faecal incontinence is usually secondary to 'overflow' to faecal retention (in 80%), it may occur without constipation (functional non-retentive fecal incontinence) in 20%. The latter is of unclear aetiology but may be associated with emotional problems.
- Hirschsprung's disease (aganglionic segment) presents with various degrees of obstruction in neonates. Empty rectum by rectal palpation may suggest disease.

Red Flags

- Constipation should not be accepted as the cause of abdominal pain without consideration of alternative diagnoses.
- Faecal incontinence associated with constipation may be mistaken as diarrhoea. The parent should receive information about mechanisms causing faecal incontinence.
- Treatment of children with faecal incontinence is urgently needed to avoid poor quality of life, poor self-esteem and social withdrawal. These features disappear after successful treatment.
- Organic causes of faecal incontinence may not be evident in every case but need to be considered in the evaluation of each case. These include tethered cord, malabsorption and endocrine causes.
- Beware that constipation may have an underlying physical, sexual or emotional cause.

FURTHER READING

Vieira MC, Negrelle ICK, Webber KU et al. Pediatrician's knowledge on the approach of functional constipation. *Rev Paul Pediatr* 2016;34(4):425–431.

DIARRHOEA

Clinical Overview

Diarrhoea is a major health problem and is the second leading cause of death among children under 5 years old, accounting for nearly half a million deaths each year globally. It is defined as three or more episodes of loose or liquid stools and/or vomiting, possibly accompanied by other symptoms such as fever, nausea and abdominal pain that results from GI inflammation. In children with vomiting alone, alternative diagnoses should be considered. Most diarrhoeal diseases in children living in developed countries are viral (75%–90% of cases), mild and self-limited, and do not require hospitalization or laboratory evaluation. Diarrhoea is usually watery, large and non-bloody. In developing countries, diarrhoea is often severe with a high rate of deaths. Frequent, small bloody stools with mucus suggest colitis. With widespread use of rotavirus vaccine beginning in 2006, a substantial decrease in disease prevalence, morbidity and mortality has been achieved. The most important aspect of evaluation of diarrhoeal case is to determine the level of dehydration.

Differential Diagnosis

Infants	Children
Common	
Physiologic in breast-fed	Acute infective enteritis, GE (viral and bacterial)
Milk protein/lactose intolerance	Antibiotic induced
Antibiotic induced	Postinfectious secondary lactose/protein intolerance
Coeliac disease	Toddler's diarrhoea
Cystic fibrosis	Overflow in constipation
Rare	
Primary disaccharide deficiency	Coeliac disease (CD)
Acrodermatitis enteropathica	IBD
Short bowel syndrome	IBS
	Malabsorption
	Nosocomial diarrhoea
	Pseudomembranous colitis (drug induced)
	Munchausen syndrome by proxy

Differential Diagnosis at a Glance

	Physiological (breast-fed)	Toddler 'Diarrhoea'	Viral GE (small bowel)	Bacterial Colitis	Milk Intolerance
Fever	No	No	Possible	Yes	No
Watery	No	No	Yes	No	Yes
Blood, mucus	No	No	No	Yes	Possible
Faecal white blood cell count	No	No	Possible	Yes	Possible
Tenesmus	No	No	No	Yes	No

Recommended Investigations

*** Stool for culture (bacterial), and antigen for viral cause (e.g. rotavirus)

**   Testing the stool with a Clinitest tablet for reducing substances to confirm lactose intolerance

**   Blood for U&E is indicated unless the diarrhoea is mild and there is little or no dehydration

Top Tips

- The principal complication from diarrhoea is dehydration. If a child is alert and playful, the degree of dehydration is insignificant.
- Mothers are usually good historians. Urine frequency and colour can give an important estimate of the degree of dehydration: concentrated urine (orange colour) suggests mild dehydration, infrequent and small amount of urine suggests moderate, and anuria means severe dehydration.
- Toddler's diarrhoea (functional diarrhoea) is the most common cause of chronic diarrhoea without failure to thrive. Excessive fruit juice and fructose consumption may play a role in the pathophysiology of this condition.
- Diarrhoea persisting for longer than 2 weeks (termed *protracted* or *chronic diarrhoea*) is mostly due to milk lactose or protein intolerance. Temporary withdrawal of milk and diary products is usually diagnostic and therapeutic.
- Large watery diarrhoea in association with diffuse abdominal pain and vomiting is typical for enteritis (usually termed *gastroenteritis*), whereas small frequent, bloody stools and lower abdominal pain are very suggestive of colitis.
- Major reduction in diarrhoea morbidity and mortality over the past decades is due to oral rehydration solution, rotavirus vaccine and zinc supplement. Probiotics may be beneficial.
- The main causes of protracted diarrhea are milk protein and lactose intolerance and CD.
- Polymer-based oral rehydration solution (ORS), using rice or wheat, has advantages over ORS <270 mOsm/L and ORS >310 mOsm/L.

Red Flags

- Beware of harmful practices in the management of diarrhoea which include restriction of fluid, breastfeeding and food and inappropriate medication use.
- Toddler's diarrhoea is common and should not be misdiagnosed as GE. These children are healthy and thriving, passing three to five soft stools daily, often containing undigested food particles (e.g. carrots, peas). It is self-limiting and resolves spontaneously when at school age.
- Children with loose, frequent stools may have an infection elsewhere, e.g. UTI or appendicitis.
- Laxative-induced diarrhoea (induced illness) is rare but should not be missed. The diarrhoea is usually chronic or recurrent. The carer of the child often has an underlying psychiatric disturbance.

FURTHER READING

Carter E, Bryce J, Perin J et al. Harmful practices in the management of childhood diarrhoea in low- and middle income countries: A systematic review. *BMC Public Health* 2015;15:788.
Greggoria GV, Gonzales MM, Dans LF et al. Polymer-based oral rehydration solution for treating acute watery diarrhoea. *Cochrane Database Syst Rev* 2016;(12):CD006519.

GASTROINTESTINAL BLEEDING (RECTAL BLEEDING)

Clinical Overview

Gastrointestinal bleeding (GIB) is a common condition and can occur from the mouth to the anus. It is classified as an upper GIB (oesophagus, stomach and duodenum) originating proximal to the ligament of Treitz (at the duodeno-jejunal junction), leading to haematemesis, coffee-ground vomiting and black tarry stools (melena). This type of GIB is uncommon in children but is potentially a life-threatening condition. Lower GIB originating from areas below the ligament of Treitz (bowel, colon) produces bright red blood that has not been in contact with gastric juice. Bright blood mixed with loose stools suggests bleeding site above the rectum (colitis, e.g. infectious or ulcerative colitis). Beyond the neonatal period, anal fissures are the most common cause of rectal bleeding. The child presents with painful defaecation and small blood streaks on the surface of the stool.

Possible Diagnoses

Infants	Children
Common	
Any cause of haematemesis	Any cause of haematemesis
Swallowed maternal blood	Bacterial colitis
Vitamin K deficiency	Anal fissure
NEC	Thrombocytopenia
Intussusception	HSP
Drugs	Colitis (e.g. ulcerative colitis)
Cow's milk protein	Meckel's diverticulum
Anal fissure	Peptic ulcer
Thrombocytopenia	Intussusception
Rare	
Volvulus	Drugs
Polyps	Peptic ulcer
Haemorrhagic diseases	Swallowed blood (e.g. from epistaxis)
Haemangioma	Oesophagitis
Oesophagitis	Haemolytic uraemic syndrome
Duplication of bowel	IBD
	Mallory–Weiss syndrome
	Hereditary haemorrhagic telangiectasia
	Angiodysplasia
	Hookworm infections

Differential Diagnosis at a Glance

	Infectious GE	Colitis	Gastric Ulcer	Intussusception	Meckel's Diverticulum
Diarrhoea	Yes	Yes	No	No	No
Massive bleed	No	No	No	No	Yes
Painless bleed	Yes	Yes	No	Yes	No
Vomiting	Yes	No	Possible	Yes	No
Bright red blood	Yes	Yes	No	Yes	Yes

Recommended Investigations

  *** Stool testing for occult blood to confirm or exclude bleeding

  *** FBC: anaemia suggests chronic blood loss; anaemia with high CRP suggests IBD; low platelets indicate thrombocytopenia

  ** Liver function tests for suspected liver disease; renal function test: high urea and creatinine suggest haemolytic-uraemic syndrome

  ** Clotting study to evaluate coagulopathies such as haemophilia

  ** Apt test to differentiate maternal from fetal blood

  *** Stool culture to confirm infective colitis

  ** Abdominal plain X-ray is useful in suspected cases of NEC and intussusception

  *** Endoscopy is indicated in GIB, also therapeutically for e.g. polyps, ulcer

Top Tips

- Rectal bleeding in a healthy neonate is most often maternal in origin, swallowed either during delivery or breastfeeding.
- Important factors in the differential diagnosis of GI bleeding: age of the child, presence or absence of anal pain during blood passage, and presence or absence of diarrhoea.
- Meckel's diverticulum should strongly be suspected at any age if bleeding is massive and accompanied by both bright and dark red stools.
- Endoscopy is the method of choice for evaluating GIB that should be performed within 24 hours of presentation, after stabilization of the child. It has also a therapeutic role for polyps and ulcers.

Red Flags

- Remember that not all red or black stools contain blood; iron, charcoal, licorice, blueberries and bismuth preparations can cause a black appearance of a stool.
- The abdominal pain in HSP may be severe and can lead to laparotomy, particularly if it precedes the skin rash and joint manifestations. Buttocks, arms and legs should be examined for urticarial lesions or petechiae.
- Children who present with persistent or recurrent iron-deficiency anaemia and occult GIB should have the stool checked for blood.

FURTHER READING

Romano C, Oliva S, Martellossi S et al. Pediatric gastrointestinal bleeding: Perspective from the Italian Society of Pediatric Gastroenterology. *World J Gastroenterol* 2017;23(8):1328–1337.

JAUNDICE

Clinical Overview

Jaundice is very common during the neonatal period: 60% of term and 80% of preterm babies become jaundiced with indirect hyperbilirubinaemia (IHB) in the first few days of life, mainly due to breakdown of red blood cells. Indirect bilirubin is fat soluble and can cause brain damage and kernicterus. After the neonatal period, infection remains the most common cause of jaundice world-wide. The viruses that causes jaundice are hepatitis A, B, C, D and E virus, cytomegalovirus, and Epstein–Barr–virus. Hepatitis A used to be a common infection, but its incidence rate has declined significantly in developed countries. It causes direct hyperbilirubinaemia (DHB). Jaundice should be differentiated from xanthochromia (carotenaemia), which is due to carotene deposits in the skin. The sclerae remain normal (Figure 2.1).

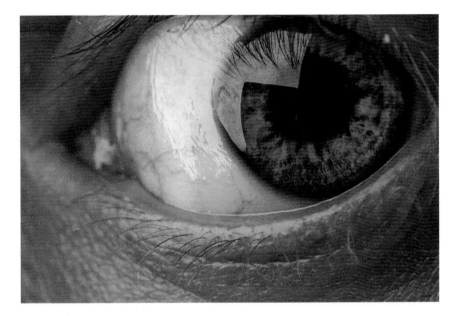

FIGURE 2.1   Sclera in patient with jaundice.

Differential Diagnosis

Infants	Children
Common	
Physiological	Infectious hepatitis
Haemolytic (ABO incompatibility)	Drug-induced jaundice
Breast milk	Mononucleosis
Polycythaemia	Haemolytic anaemia
Parenteral hyperalimentation	Gilbert syndrome
Rare	
Congenital spherocytosis	Malaria
Congenital hepatitis, cytomegalovirus (CMV), rubella	Reye syndrome
Toxoplasmosis, syphilis	Autoimmune liver disease

(Continued)

(Continued)

Infants	Children
Biliary atresia	Wilson disease
Hypothyroidism	Yellow fever
Metabolic (e.g. galactosaemia)	Cystic fibrosis
Niemann-Pick disease	Liver cirrhosis
Alagille syndrome	Crigler-Najjar syndrome
α-1 Antitrypsin deficiency	Lyme disease
Cystic fibrosis	Q fever
	Leptospirosis
	Choledochal cyst
	Typhoid fever
	Wilson disease
	Hepatic abscess
	Niemann-Pick disease

Differential Diagnosis at a Glance

	Infectious Hepatitis	Drug Induced	Mononucleosis	Gilbert Syndrome	Haemolytic Anaemia
Fever	Yes	Possible	Yes	Possible	Possible
Anaemia	No	Possible	No	No	Yes
Splenomegaly	Possible	No	Yes	No	Possible
Lymphadenopathy	Possible	No	Yes	No	No
Abdominal pain	Yes	Possible	Possible	Yes	Possible

Recommended Investigations

*** FBC: Hb low in haemolysis; leukocytosis suggests infection; reticulocytosis suggests haemolysis

*** Liver functions tests should include total bilirubin and direct bilirubin (for persistent jaundice longer than 2 weeks), alkaline phosphatase, prothrombin time (PT), partial thromboplastin time (PTT), albumin

*** Blood group and Rh-status of the mother and infant, Coombs test

** Tests for intrauterine infections (TORCH)

** Thyroid function tests to assess thyroid function

*** Abdominal ultrasound scan: to rule out bile obstruction (e.g. choledochal cyst)

** Isotope scan with technetium; percutaneous needle liver biopsy may occasionally be indicated

Top Tips

- Physiologic jaundice occurs in most neonates during the first few days of life: it is not a disease, it is not present in the first 24 hours, and it is always an IHB.
- Breast milk jaundice is physiologic jaundice, which may persist for weeks in about 10% of breastfed babies. Mothers should be encouraged to continue breastfeeding.
- An infant or toddler with yellow skin but normal white sclera has carotenaemia, not jaundice.
- Direct-reacting bilirubin is water soluble, not fat soluble, and therefore does not damage the brain tissue to cause kernicterus. It is, however, associated with serious diseases, such as congenital hepatitis and biliary atresia.
- In hepatocellular disease, there is a disproportional increase of alanine aminotransferase (ALT) and aspartate aminotransferase (AST) compared to alkaline phosphatase increase;

whereas in cholestatic diseases it is the opposite. ALT is present in the liver, hence more specific than AST which is present in other organs.

- A healthy full-term baby without haemolysis will not get any ill effect from a bilirubin <400 μmol.
- Gilbert syndrome is the most common cause of indirect bilirubin jaundice in older children. It is a benign condition; patients are usually asymptomatic. Jaundice becomes apparent during fasting or stress. It should be differentiated from haemolytic disease (by Hb, reticulocyte count).
- Although hepatitis is the most common cause of jaundice worldwide, jaundice occurs in as few as 1 in 10 children with hepatitis A, 1 in 4 with hepatitis B, and in less than 1 in 3 with hepatitis C.

Red Flags

- Always measure serum bilirubin in babies with jaundice in the first 24 hours of life.
- Children with acute UTI present occasionally with jaundice that may divert attention to hepatic disease, causing delay in antibiotic administration. The infection can progress to septicaemia.
- Be aware that children with biliary atresia are usually healthy looking and indistinguishable from those with physiological jaundice during the first 2 weeks.
- When jaundice lasts more than more than 2 weeks, always measure direct bilirubin and ask for 'pale chalky' stools and/or dark urine that stain the nappy. These are suggestive of biliary atresia. Absence of pale stools does not always exclude biliary atresia.
- Direct bilirubin more than 25 μmol/L (or 15% of the total bilirubin) indicates serious disease and is never physiologic. Causes include neonatal hepatitis secondary to congenital infection (rubella, CMV, toxoplasmosis) or biliary atresia.
- It is vitally important to refer an infant with DHB as an emergency before irreversible damage to the liver is done. The Kasai operation (portoenterostomy) is successful (>90%) if performed before 8 weeks of life. Without Kasai operation (to drain bile from the liver into the intestines) or liver transplantation, liver failure ensues within a year and death within 2 years.

FURTHER READING

Wang KS. Newborn screening for biliary atresia. *Pediatrics* 2015;136(6):e1663–e1669.

VOMITING

Clinical Overview

Vomiting is included in the recent terminology of functional gastrointestinal disorders (FGIDs), which are chronic or refractory symptoms without structural or biochemical abnormalities. These include infant regurgitation, infant colic, cyclic vomiting and functional nausea and vomiting. Vomiting is a forceful action accomplished by a downward contraction of the diaphragm, along with tightening of the abdominal muscles against an open sphincter, propelling gastric contents out. Unlike vomiting, regurgitation indicates discharge of gastric contents without effort and nausea. Retching signals the beginning of vomiting. These steps are coordinated by the medullary vomiting centre, which receives afferent signals from the GI tract, bloodstream, equilibrium system of the inner ear and central nervous system (CNS). Because vomiting is a common symptom in children, it should be evaluated in the clinical context with other associated symptoms. Clinicians should be in a position to determine the degree of seriousness of vomiting. In this section, only vomiting as a major symptom is discussed.

Possible Diagnoses

Infants	Children
Common	
GO reflux	Gastroenteritis
Swallowed blood or fluid during delivery	Systemic infection (e.g. pneumonia, UTI)
Systemic infection	Medications (e.g. chemotherapy)
Intestinal obstruction	GO reflux
Pyloric stenosis	Migraine
Rare	
Overfeeding	Appendicitis
Overfeeding (mainly in prematurity)	Meningitis
Milk protein/lactose intolerance	Postoperative
Inborn errors of metabolism (e.g. galactosaemia)	Periodic syndrome (cyclic vomiting)
Sepsis	Intestinal obstruction
Oesophageal atresia	Increased intracranial pressure (CNS tumour)
Intussusception	Pertussis
Subdural haematoma	IBD
Rumination	Peptic ulcer
Cyclic vomiting	Eating disorders (bulimia)
	Norovirus
	Head injury
	Pancreatitis
	Inborn errors of metabolism
	Renal or biliary colic

Differential Diagnosis at a Glance

	Gastroenteritis	Systemic Infections	GO Reflux	Migraine	Medication
Diarrhoea	Yes	Possible	No	No	Possible
Positive family history	Possible	No	No	Yes	No
Thriving	Possible	Yes	Possible	Yes	Yes
With fever	Possible	Yes	No	No	No
Acute onset	Yes	Yes	No	Yes	Yes

Recommended Investigations

Investigation should be directed according to the history and clinical findings.

** Urine for reducing substance for suspected galactosaemia
** Blood for FBC, CRP, U&E for persistent vomiting
** Blood glucose, blood gases, amino acids, lactate, carnitine for inborn errors of metabolism
** Abdominal and chest X-ray is useful in intestinal obstruction
** Abdominal ultrasound scan to confirm cases of pyloric stenosis

Top Tips

- GO reflux is common in infants and refers to the involuntary passage of gastric contents into the oesophagus, which is a normal phenomenon occurring many times a day in both children and adults. Reflux occurs commonly in infants because of liquid milk-based diet, recumbent position and immaturity of the GO junction.
- Norovirus is a common cause of vomiting and gastroenteritis (GE). After the introduction of rotavirus vaccines, norovirus is the leading cause of GE in children younger than 5 years of age.
- The vast majority of infants with GO reflux do well aged 6–12 months; few develop complications including oesophagitis, aspiration pneumonia and abnormal neck and head posturing (Sandifer syndrome). The condition is then termed GO reflux disease.
- Pyloric stenosis is differentiated from GO reflux by projectile vomiting in the first 2–3 weeks of life in a baby who is hungry with visible gastric peristalsis and a palpation of an 'olive' in the right upper quadrant. With reflux, children vomit during or immediately after feeding.
- Once a pyloric tumour is palpated in the abdomen (present in about 50% of cases), this is pathognomonic for the disease. If in doubt, an ultrasound is a very useful tool in experienced hands. A thickness of >4 mm suggests the diagnosis.
- Cyclic vomiting is characterised by current (three attacks in 6 months or five attacks in any time) vomiting with symptom-free intervals. A family history of migraine supports the diagnosis.
- Anti-emetics are rarely used in paediatrics; finding the underlying cause of the vomiting is far more important than spending time selecting an anti-emetic. Exceptions include chemotherapy-induced vomiting and persistent vomiting in migraine.

Red Flags

- Although dehydration is the main complication of vomiting, particularly in infants and young children, hypochloraemic hypokalaemic alkalosis and bleeding from tears in the distal oesophagus may occur with recurrent forceful vomiting.
- Bilious vomiting may occur after an hour or two after any repeated vomiting and retching, but it usually suggests intestinal obstruction requiring immediate medical attention.
- Beware that pain usually precedes vomiting in appendicitis and intestinal obstruction.
- Not all vomiting with headache is migraine; a CNS lesion such as brain tumour must be excluded.
- Vomiting causes metabolic alkalosis; vomiting causing metabolic acidosis is suggestive of gastroenteritis or inborn error of metabolism.
- Cyclic vomiting (CV) is often misdiagnosed as gastroenteritis or GO reflux. Conditions mimicking CV include mitochondrial disorders, fatty acid oxidation disorder and organic aciduria. Elevated lactate and metabolic acidosis are important clues.
- Consider inborn errors of metabolism in the differential diagnosis of any severely ill neonate who presents with poor feeding, lethargy, vomiting and convulsion in early life. The condition is often lethal unless prompt treatment is initiated.

FURTHER READING

Chow S, Goldman RD. Treating children cyclic vomiting. *Can Fam Physician* 2007;53(3):417–419.

VOMITING BLOOD (HAEMATEMESIS)

Clinical Overview

GIB may originate anywhere from the mouth to the anus. Upper gastrointestinal bleeding (UGIB) is much less common in children than in adults because of rarity of GI cancers. Haematemesis, with or without melaena, usually indicates a bleed from a site proximal to the ligament of Treitz of the duodenum (duodeno-jejunal junction). Haematochezia refers to distal bleeding. When haematemesis is caused by brisk bleeding, it usually indicates an arterial source. Coffee-ground emesis results from blood altered by gastric acid and usually means that the bleeding has slowed or stopped. The causes of haematemesis vary according to the age of the child and whether there are other associated symptoms. Haematemesis (usually associated with nausea, act of vomiting, pain and possible tenderness of the abdomen) must be differentiated from haemoptysis (associated with cough, frothy colour, crackle noises on lung auscultation and evidence of pulmonary disease) and swallowed epistaxis (blood present in the nose, dripping into the posterior nasopharynx).

Possible Diagnoses

Infants	Children
Common	
Swallowed maternal blood (during birth)	Drugs
Swallowed blood from cracked nipple	Gastritis
Oesophagitis secondary to GO reflux	Mallory–Weiss tear (MWT)
NEC	Oesophagitis (GO reflux)
Blood disorders (e.g. thrombocytopenia)	Swallowed blood (e.g. epistaxis)
Rare	
Coagulation disorder	Oesophageal varices (usually large haematemesis)
DIC	Gastric erosion or ulcer
Meckel's diverticulum	Thrombocytopenia
Haemophilia	Swallowing of foreign body
	Gastric vascular malformation
	Haemophilia
	Gastric tumour

Differential Diagnosis at a Glance

	Drugs	Gastritis	MWT	GO Reflux	Swallowed Blood
Associated pain	Possible	Yes	Possible	Yes	No
Preceded by vomiting	Possible	Possible	Yes	Yes	No
Prior severe retching	No	No	Yes	No	No
Massive bleeding	Possible	Possible	Yes	No	No
Affects infancy	Possible	Possible	No	Yes	No

Recommended Investigations

*** FBC: anaemia suggests chronic blood loss or large blood loss; thrombocytopenia

*** Coagulation studies: PT, PTT, clotting factors and LFTs

*** Apt test: maternal (blood turns yellow-brown) or fetal: blood remains pink

*** Abdominal plain X-ray useful for NEC, or foreign body
*** Abdominal ultrasound scan for suspected intussusception
*** Endoscopy for upper GI bleed

Tip Tops

- In haematemesis, the history usually suggests the likely diagnosis and tests are often not required.
- Causes of haematemesis are age dependent: in neonates it is mostly caused by swallowed maternal blood; in infancy it is mostly caused by drugs or reflux oesophagitis; in older children it is mostly caused by drugs, MWT, oesophageal varices (portal hypertension) or peptic ulcer.
- UGIB may present with haematemesis alone, with melaena alone or a combination of both.
- MWT was described in 1929 in association with alcohol bingeing; it is not that common in children. GO reflux remains one of the most common causes of this tear.
- In a baby with haematemesis, inspection of the mother's breast or expressed milk suggests the diagnosis, and it is confirmed by Apt-test performed on blood aspirated from the stomach.
- Vomiting blood may be bright red or dark and resemble coffee grounds; the latter indicates digestion of blood by gastric juice.

Red Flags

- Stabilisation of the child with open airway and blood transfusion is urgent. The child may rapidly deteriorate, leading to circulatory collapse.
- When a newborn has haematemesis or melaena, consider if he or she was not given vitamin K.
- Haemoglobin on admission may not reflect the true haemoglobin level or the blood loss, and therefore frequent Hb check is recommended.
- Haematemesis caused by medications, particularly non-steroidal anti-inflammatory drugs (NSAIDs), is underreported and underestimated; it is always worth taking a detailed history of recent intake of drugs. The condition is often misdiagnosed as 'viral gastritis'.
- Aspirin should not be given to children (except in certain indications, e.g. Kawasaki disease). Parents may not be aware that many over-the-counter cough remedies and analgesics contain aspirin.
- MWT (linear laceration at the GO junction) may occur after a single episode of vomiting. Children with portal hypertension are at high risk of this tear.

FURTHER READING

Nasher O, Devadason D, Stewart RJ et al. Upper gastrointestinal bleeding in children: A tertiary United Kingdom children's hospital experience. *Children (Basel).* 4(11), 2017. doi:10.3390/children4110095

3 SYSTEMIC PHYSICAL CONDITION

CRYING, EXCESSIVE (INCLUDING BABY COLIC)

Clinical Overview

When crying is inconsolable and excessive, it can cause stress to parents, disrupt parenting and, in rare cases, place an infant at risk for abuse. It is common and normal for infants to cry up to 2 hours a day. Infantile colic is not a diagnosis; it is simply a term that describes healthy infants with paroxysmal excessive crying for no apparent reason, presumably of intestinal origin, during the first 3–4 months. It is defined as crying for over 3 hours a day, over 3 days a week and over 3 weeks. It usually begins aged 2 weeks and significantly improves by the age of 3–4 months. Characteristically, the attack begins suddenly, is continuous, with flushed face, tense abdomen, hands making fists and drawing up of legs. Around 5% of cases have organic causes. Crying may be a baby's way of communication; as children grow older, they find different ways to communicate.

Possible Diagnoses

Infants	Children
Common	
Colic (evening colic)	Pain (e.g. abdominal pain)
Discomfort (too warm or too cold, nappy rash)	Food intolerance (including milk intolerance)
Gastro-oesophageal (GO) reflux	GO reflux
Infection (e.g. otitis media [OM])	Infection (e.g. OM)
Milk and food allergy/intolerance	Night terror
Rare	
Non-accidental injury	Non-accidental injury
Intestinal obstruction (e.g. intussusception)	Intestinal obstruction (e.g. intussusception)
Constipation	Renal stones or gallstone
Teething	Migraine
Maternal migraine	

Differential Diagnosis at a Glance

	Colic	GO Reflux	Food Intolerance	Infection	Night Terror
Short history	No	No	Possible	Yes	No
Associated vomiting	No	Yes	Possible	No	No
Within 6 months of age	Yes	Yes	Possible	No	No
Symptoms mainly evening	Yes	No	No	No	Yes
Effective therapy available	No	Yes	Yes	Yes	No

Recommended Investigations

The following tests are sometimes required:

*** Urinalysis to exclude urinary tract infection (UTI)
**   Full blood count (FBC) and C-reactive protein (CRP) for infection such as appendicitis
*** Plain X-ray of abdomen for intestinal obstruction, e.g. intussusception
*** Abdominal ultrasound scan for renal or gallbladder stone intestinal obstruction
**   pH study to confirm GO reflux

Top Tips

- Colic typically is noted more in the afternoon and evening (commonly 6–10 P.M.), suggesting that events at home (e.g. parent is busy with household; child being left alone) could be the major cause. Evening colic used to be the most common diagnosis of infantile colic; this is being replaced by GO reflux.
- Persistent crying beyond 4 months of age has been associated with long-term psychological and behavioural problems, including hyperactivity and migraine.
- GO reflux is considered physiological when the infant thrives with some posseting/vomiting. When GO reflux is causing complications, e.g. irritability, disrupted sleep, choking, aspiration pneumonia and/or poor weight gain, it is termed *GO reflux disease.*
- Although several over-the-counter preparations are used for colic (gripe water, Infacol, Dentinox), they are scientifically not proven.
- A sympathetic and supportive clinician who has time to listen to parental concerns of excessive crying is a prerequisite for successful management.
- Sedation or temporary hospital admission is occasionally required for babies with excessive crying. This is done if other measures fail and often for a maternal indication, i.e. to give relief to an exhausted mother.

Red Flags

- The diagnosis of colic should not be made without excluding more serious disorders such as otitis media or intussusception.
- A child who develops severe paroxysmal abdominal pain after the age of 3–4 months should be examined to exclude organic causes, e.g. UTI or intussusception.
- Beware that the fontanelle can be bulging when the baby is crying; if it remains so after cessation of crying, this sign is serious and occurs in meningitis or hydrocephalus.
- The administration of a sedative to a child with persistent crying may mask an underlying abdominal pathology; it should be the last resort.
- Be aware of the possibility of non-accidental injury for unexplained baby crying. Check the baby's weight (failure to thrive?); check for any bruises in the skin.
- Early increase in crying in a healthy infant is the most common stimulus for shaken baby syndrome (abusive head trauma). This is a potentially lethal form of physical abuse causing brain injury, e.g. subdural haematoma, with 80% significant brain injury and 20% death.

FURTHER READING

Barr RG. Preventing abusive head trauma resulting from a failure of normal interaction between infants and their caregivers. *Proc Natl Acad Sci USA* 2012;109(Suppl 2):17294–17301.

Dahlen HG, Foster JP, Psalia K et al. Gastro-oesophageal reflux: A mixed methods study of infants admitted to hospital in the first 12 months following birth in NSW. *BMC Pediatr* 2018;18:30.

Zeevenhooven J, Koppen IJN, Benninga MA. The new Rome IV criteria for functional gastrointestinal disorders in infants and toddlers. *Pediatr Gastroenterol Hepatol Nutr* 2017;20(1):1–13.

FAILURE TO THRIVE AND WEIGHT LOSS

Clinical Overview

Although there is no agreement about a definition of failure to thrive (FTT), a child whose weight is well below the third percentile (or more accurately if the weight is below 0.4 percentile on the 9 percentile chart) or a weight loss that has crossed two percentiles should be considered as FTT. It is a descriptive term, not a diagnosis, with peak incidence occurring in children 1–2 years of age. FFT is divided into two main categories: organic and non-organic causes. Globally, malnutrition/under-nutrition is the most common cause of FTT. In children living in high-income countries, psychosocial causes are far more common than organic causes. If the history and physical examination do not suggest a specific underlying organic disease, psychosocial causes are likely and laboratory tests and imaging are unlikely to provide the answer.

Possible Diagnoses

Infants	Children
Common	
Small for date	Psychosocial (e.g. emotional deprivation)
Neglect	Eating disorder (e.g. anorexia nervosa)
Milk allergy	Chronic infection (e.g. HIV, parasitic)
Malnutrition	Malnutrition and under-nutrition (from poverty)
Malabsorption	Malabsorption (e.g. coeliac disease)
Rare	
GO reflux	Malignancy
Inborn errors of metabolism	Depression, anxiety
Chronic diarrhoea	Inflammatory bowel diseases
Prematurity	GO reflux
Chronic diseases	Induced illness (Munchausen by proxy)
CNS tumour	Inborn errors of metabolism
	CNS tumour

Differential Diagnosis at a Glance

	Psychological (Neglect)	Eating Disorder	Chronic Infections	Malnutrition	Malabsorption
Diagnostic history	Yes	Possible	Possible	Yes	Yes
Peak 1–2 years of age	Yes	No	Possible	Yes	Yes
Abnormal stools	No	No	Possible	Possible	Yes
Abnormal physical examination	No	No	Possible	Yes	Yes
Reduced activity	Possible	Possible	Possible	Possible	No

Recommended Investigations

***   Urine: proteinuria in renal disease
***   FBC: Low haemoglobin suggests anaemia in malnutrition, infection and malabsorption
**   Serum albumin
**   Inflammatory markers (CRP or erythrocyte sedimentation rate [ESR]): elevated in infectious diseases

*** TFTs will confirm hyperthyroidism
*** Coeliac screening tests in blood
*** Consider cranial MRI if no cause for weight loss has been identified

Top Tips

- Small-for-gestational-age babies (weight less than the 10th percentile for gestational age) dated from the first trimester (symmetrically affecting the height and head circumference [HC] as well) often remain underweight. They should not be categorised as FTT.
- Malabsorption is characterised by diarrhoea of greater than four stools a day and/or steatorrhoea, i.e., fat content in stool >4 g a day for infant, and >6–8 g in older children.
- Neglect, whether nutritional or emotional, is the most common cause of underweight in infancy and may account for more than 50% of cases with FTT.
- Community paediatricians have a central role in the care of children with chronic illness and in supporting their families. The main role of paediatricians is establishing a diagnosis and arranging referrals to subspecialties and other medical facilities.
- Depressive disorder is not uncommon in adolescents, who may show either a decrease or an increase in weight.

Red Flags

- Children who were small for their gestational age often have slow weight gain during the first 1–3 years of life. They have to be differentiated from those who have gained weight and then experience weight loss. The latter group should be taken very seriously.
- Be aware of children at a high risk of abuse: excessive crying during infancy, physical handicap, chronic illness, with behavioural or learning difficulties.
- Early detection of psychosocial problems (e.g. neglect) is very important because it can result not only in poor physical growth but also in poor cognitive and intellectual development.
- Neglected children returning to their parents without any medical or social intervention may face serious re-injury (in about 25%) or death (in about 5%).
- Weight loss in adolescent girls is likely to be due to eating disorder. Diagnosis can be difficult in the early stages. Asking about attitude toward eating and weight will suggest the diagnosis.

FURTHER READING

Ross E, Munoz FM, Edem B et al. Failure to thrive: Case definition and guidelines for data collection, analysis and presentation of maternal immunisation safety data. *Vaccine* 2017;35(48):6483–6491.

Rudolf M, Logan S. What is the long term outcome for children who fail to thrive? A systematic review. *Arch Dis Child* 2005;90(9):925–931.

POSTOPERATIVE FEVER

Clinician Overview

Postoperative fever is defined as a temperature greater than 38°C on two consecutive postoperative days, or 39°C on any postoperative day. Fever during the postoperative period is common, occurring in 25%–50% of cases. The magnitude of fever is correlated with the extent of the surgery, i.e. minor surgery is rarely associated with fever. Early postoperative fever (within 48 hours postoperatively) is often caused by the trauma of the surgery. Infection is the cause of fever in about 10%–25% of febrile postoperative patients, usually occurring after 48 hours. Fever usually lasts longer than 2 days (unless treated with antibiotics) tends to be higher than 39°C, and is associated with ill appearance.

Possible Diagnoses

Infants	Children
Common	
Dehydration	Dehydration
High ambient temperature	Wound infection
Septicaemia	Transfusion or drug reaction
Intravenous line infection	Haematoma
Haematoma	Pneumonia
Rare	
Infectious diarrhoea	Haematoma
Urinary tract infection (UTI)	UTI
Osteomyelitis	Bacteraemia
Pulmonary atelectasis	

Differential Diagnosis at a Glance

	Dehydration	Wound infection	Transfusion/ drug reaction	Haematoma	Pneumonia
High fever	No	Possible	No	No	Yes
Fever on day one of surgery	Yes	No	Yes	No	No
Ill appearance	Yes	Possible	Possible	No	Yes
Diagnosis by seeing surgical site	No	Yes	No	Yes	No
Leukocytosis & high CRP	No	Yes	Possible	Possible	Yes

Recommended Investigation

- ** Urine culture
- *** Full blood count
- ** Liver function tests
- *** Blood culture
- ** Chest X-ray
- ** Viral studies: occasionally requested if the fever persists
- ** CT scan and/or ultrasonography: sometimes required for detecting intra-abdominal abscess

Top Tips

- Physical examination should focus on sites most likely to be the cause of fever, including the operative site, abdomen (for distension, tenderness, absence of bowel sounds) and upper respiratory tract for infection and lung auscultation.
- The diagnosis of non-infectious causes should only be considered after excluding infectious causes.
- Factors that increase the likelihood of infection include long postoperative stay in hospital, fever commencing on the third postoperative day or later and fever over 39°C that persists or has a hectic pattern, and the presence of intravascular catheter, the prolonged use of naso-gastric or endotracheal tube, indwelling urinary catheter or shunt.

Red Flags

- Beware that serious infection may exist in the absence of fever; this is usually the case during the neonatal period and in immunosuppressed children.
- The importance of postoperative fever exists in the possibility of infection, which can lead to death if not properly treated.
- Although most postoperative fevers are non-infectious, patients should be treated with antibiotics if they appear unwell, the source of the fever is obscured or there is leukocytosis with high CRP.
- Before embarking on performing tests for postoperative fever, remember that the most common source of infectious fever is wound infection.

FURTHER READING

Gupta AK, Singh VK, Varma A. Approach to postoperative fever in pediatric cardiac patients. *Ann Pediatr Cardiol* 2012;5(1):61–68.

RECURRENT FEVER (PERIODIC AND RELAPSING FEVER)

Clinician Overview

Periodic fever (PF) and relapsing fever (ReF) are characterized by episodes of fever recurring at regular or irregular intervals; each episode is followed by one to several days, weeks or months of normal temperature. Examples are seen in malaria, brucellosis, familial Mediterranean fever (FMF) and PFAPA (periodic fever, aphthous stomatitis, pharyngitis, and cervical adenitis). ReF is recurrent fever caused by numerous species of Borrelia and transmitted by lice (louse-borne ReF) or ticks (tick-borne ReF). Familial cold urticaria syndrome (FCUS), Muckle–Wells syndrome (MWS), TNF-receptor associated periodic syndrome (TRAPS) and hyperimmunoglobulinemia D syndrome (HIDS) are also characterized by recurrent episodes of fever but they are rare compared with FMF.

Possible Diagnoses

Infants	Children
Common	
FMF	Malaria
Brucellosis	Brucellosis
Malaria	FMF
MWS	PFAPA
Cyclic neutropenia	Cyclic neutropenia
Rare	
FCUS	FCUS
	TRAPS
	MWS
	HIDS

Differential Diagnosis at a Glance

	Malaria	Brucellosis	FMF	PFAPA	Cyclic neutropenia
Inheritance	No	No	Yes	Yes	Yes
Periodic fever 3–6 weeks	No	No	Yes	Yes	Yes
Mouth ulcers	No	No	No	Yes	Yes
Myalgia/arthralgia	Yes	Yes	Yes	No	No
Prevalent in Mediterranean area	Possible	Yes	Yes	No	No

Recommended Investigation

*** FBC: neutropenia < 1000 will confirm cyclic neutropenia.

*** IgD is elevated in HIDS and in the majority of cases of PFAPA.

*** Giemsa-stained smear for malaria, serological test for brucellosis.

** CRP and ESR: usually elevated.

Top Tips

- Genetic causes of periodic fever syndromes have been identified in the past few years. The term auto-inflammatory disease has been proposed to describe a group of disorders characterized by attacks of unprovoked systemic inflammation without significant levels of autoimmune or infective causes.
- FMF occurs in individuals from Mediterranean ancestry who usually present with loss of appetite and abdominal pain due to peritonitis. About 6–10 hours later, fever occurs and rapid recovery ensues within 24–72 hours.
- Pel–Ebstein fever was originally thought to be characteristic of Hodgkin's lymphoma (HL). Only a few patients with Hodgkin's disease develop this pattern, but when present, it is suggestive of HD. The pattern consists of recurrent episodes of fever lasting 3–10 days, followed by an afebrile period of similar duration.
- Episodes of fever, aphthous stomatitis, pharyngitis and cervical adenopathy (PFAPA) are the most common clinical features of auto-inflammatory disease. Each episode is followed by a symptom-free interval ranging from weeks to months.
- Patients with FMF usually respond dramatically to colchicine at 0.6 mg hourly for 4 doses, which is also effective in preventing attacks of FMF and the development of amyloidosis. For those with PFAPA, steroid therapy is very effective in controlling fever and other symptoms within 2–4 hours. Immunoglobulin-D (IgD) is elevated in the majority of cases of PFAPA.

Red Flags

- Amyloidosis commonly complicates FMF. Proteinuria is often the clue of the disease. The best site to confirm the diagnosis is biopsy from the gingiva or rectum, not from kidney or spleen.
- Cyclic neutropenia, autosomal dominant, is characterized by pharyngitis, mouth ulcers and lymphadenitis. It is easily diagnosed by recognizing the periodicity of symptoms and neutropenia.
- The resolution of febrile episode in periodic fever may be accompanied within a few hours (6–8 hours) by the Jarisch–Herxheimer reaction (JHR), which usually follows antibiotic treatment. The reaction is caused by the release of endotoxin when the organisms are destroyed by antibiotics. JHR is very common after treating patients with syphilis.

FURTHER READING

Soon GS, Laxer RM. Approach to recurrent fever in childhood. *Can Fam Physician* 2017;63(10):756–762.

TIREDNESS/FATIGUE

Clinical Overview

Everyone experiences fatigue, but recovery is rapid following a rest or a good sleep. Most childhood diseases, particularly infections, cause fatigue, which may last for many days and sometimes weeks. Chronic fatigue syndrome (CFS) is defined as an unexplained, persistent and overwhelming tiredness, weakness or exhaustion causing disruption of daily life and resulting in a decrease of physical and/or mental work, unrelieved by sleep. The condition typically exacerbates with exercise or physical activity. A minimum of 3 months is required before diagnosis is made. CFS is rare before the age of 10 years.

Possible Diagnoses

Infants	Children
Common	
Chronic respiratory diseases	CFS
Cardiac diseases	Post-viral fatigue
Drugs (e.g. anti-epileptics)	Drugs (e.g. antihistamine, anti-epileptics)
Neuromuscular diseases	Psychiatric illness (e.g. depression, anxiety disorder)
Chronic infection/inflammation	Trauma (post-traumatic stress, child abuse)
Rare	
Malnutrition/chronic anaemia	Autoimmune disease, for example, juvenile idiopathic arthritis (JIA)
Botulism	Neuromuscular diseases (e.g. myasthenia gravis)
Malignancy	Obstructive sleep apnoea
Obstructive sleep apnoea	Chronic infectious/inflammatory diseases
Hypokalaemia	Malnutrition/chronic anaemia
	Endocrine disorders (e.g. Addison's, hypothyroidism)
	Malignancy (e.g. lymphoma, neuroblastoma)
	Fibromyalgia
	Inflammatory bowel diseases (e.g. Crohn's disease)
	HIV infection
	Hypokalaemia

Differential Diagnosis at a Glance

	CFS	Post-Viral	Drugs	Psychiatric	Trauma
Preceded by viral infection	Possible	Yes	No	No	No
Fatigue as the main symptom	Yes	Yes	No	No	No
Symptoms longer than 3 months	Yes	No	No	No	No
Rest relieves fatigue	No	Possible	Yes	Possible	Possible
Normal physical examination	Possible	Possible	Possible	Yes	Yes

Recommended Investigations

*** Urine: for renal abnormalities, for example, chronic renal failure and tubular acidosis

*** FBC: Haemoglobin for chronic anaemia and infection; white blood cell (WBC) count for infection

*** U&E: in renal failure and hypokalaemia
*** Liver function tests (LFTs) for chronic infection, jaundice, anaemia
*** TFTs to confirm hypothyroidism, cortisol level for suspected Addison's disease
*** Creatine phosphokinase for suspected muscle disease
*** Serology for coeliac disease, toxoplasmosis, Lyme disease
** Serological or polymerase chain reaction studies for cytomegalovirus, EBV, Toxoplasma gondii
*** IgM for toxoplasmosis, Epstein–Barr virus (EBV), cytomegalovirus (CMV)
** Viral tests for EBV-IgM and IgG
*** Mantoux test for suspected tuberculosis (TB)
*** Chest X-ray for suspected lymphoma

Top Tips

- CFS should be differentiated from post-viral fatigue; the latter is of short duration. A history of a viral infection at onset and laboratory evidence support the diagnosis of post-viral fatigue.
- Children with autoimmune diseases (e.g. JIA or SLE) commonly suffer from fatigue for months and years even after the disease has settled.
- Childhood trauma causes sometimes a long-term fatigue. Trauma is defined as exposure to actual or threatening death, serious injury or sexual violence. This includes experiencing a direct trauma, witnessing it or learning about it.
- While fibromyalgia is characterised by widespread musculoskeletal pain (generalised or localised), joint tenderness and to a lesser extent fatigue, in CFS the fatigue is prominent, overshadowing other symptoms.
- In myasthenia gravis, the fatigue is characteristically late in the day or after exercise; ptosis is a typical presentation.
- CFS can be an extremely isolating illness. Establishing contacts with a support group can be very helpful for overcoming isolation and providing contact with similar-aged patients. A child is best managed in CFS centres, which are led by CFS specialists.

Red Flags

- Diagnosis of CFS should not be made in patients with prior history of depressive or psychotic disorder such as schizophrenia.
- Patients with CSF have often sleep disturbance; a good history of the sleep pattern is essential.
- Be aware that one of the most common and distressing side effects of cancer treatment is fatigue, occurring in up to 99% of cases. Aerobic exercise, physical activity and yoga are beneficial, not prescribing psychostimulants.
- Childhood trauma that includes sexual violence and maltreatment (physical, emotional and neglect) has detrimental effects on the cognitive and brain development of the child. Only 22% of children who had been abused or neglected achieved healthy adult functioning.

FURTHER READING

De Bellis MD, Zisk A. The biological effects of childhood trauma. *Child Adolesc Psychiatr Clin N Am* 2014;23(2):185–222.
Rowe PC, Ra U, Friedman KJ et al. Myalgic encephalomyelitis/chronic fatigue syndrome diagnosis and management in young people: A primer. *Front Pediatr* 2017;5:121.

UNEXPLAINED AND PERSISTENT FEVER

Clinical Overview

Fever without focus (FWF) is defined as an acute febrile illness without apparent source that lasts for less than a week, with the history and physical examination failing to find the cause. About 20% of all febrile episodes demonstrate no localising signs on presentation. The most common cause is a viral infection that should be considered only after excluding UTI and bacteraemia. Persistent fever (pyrexia) of unknown origin (PUO) is defined as fever without localising signs that persists for over 1 week during which evaluation fails to detect the cause. Infections are the most common causes, accounting for 60%–70% of all cases, of which about 15% are due to viral infection. Collagen diseases account for about 20%, of which the most common cause is JIA as a pre-arthritic presentation. Malignancy presenting as fever without other manifestations may occur in up to 5%. Miscellaneous diagnoses account for 5%–10% and undiagnosed in the remaining 5%. Previously, a high percentage of PUO (up to 25%) was categorised as undiagnosed, but the percentage of undiagnosed cases has greatly decreased.

Possible Diagnoses

Infants	Children
Common	
Maternal fever	Viral infection (e.g. Human herpesvirus 6 [HHV-6])
Viral infection	UTI
UTI	Occult bacteraemia
Occult bacteraemia	Collagen diseases (e.g. JIA, SLE)
Occult abscess	Parasitic infections (e.g. malaria, Lyme disease)
Rare	
Drug fever	Drug fever
Malaria	Sinusitis
Periodic and relapsing fever	Periodic and relapsing fever
Occult abscess	Occult abscess
Meningitis	Dengue fever
Anhidrotic ectodermal dysplasia	Subacute thyroiditis (de Quervain's disease)
	Neoplasms
	Inflammatory bowel disease

Differential Diagnosis at a Glance

	Viral Infection	UTI	Bacteraemia	Collagen Disease	Parasitic Infection
Well appearing	Yes	Possible	Possible	Yes	Possible
Fever 38°C–39°C	Yes	Possible	No	No	Possible
Persists longer than 1 week	No	No	No	Yes	Yes
More prevalent in females than in males	No	Yes	No	Yes	No
High WBC, CRP	No	Yes	Yes	Possible	Possible

Recommended Investigations

*** Urine: dipsticks may show positive nitrite that is highly sensitive for UTI
*** FBC: leukocytosis and high CRP suggest bacterial infection, e.g. bacteraemia or UTI
*** BC: for highly febrile children (>39°C)
*** Anti-nuclear antibodies: for autoimmune diseases such as juvenile idiopathic arthritis (JIA)
** LFTs, serum albumin: globulin ratio
*** Thick and thin peripheral film for suspected malaria
** Abdominal ultrasound scan looking for any hidden abscess in case of PUO
*** Tuberculin test
** Chest X-ray for possible TB; CT scan for sinuses
** Echocardiography for vegetation in endocarditis
** Isotope bone scan: to look for any osteomyelitic focus or tumour
** Virological studies, including polymerase chain reaction testing
** Serology for brucellosis, toxoplasmosis, CMV, EBV, salmonella

Top Tips

- Children with a viral infection are likely to appear well, with good eye contact, a reasonable level of activity, not dehydrated, and eating and drinking satisfactorily.
- Exanthema subitum (caused by HH-6; Figure 3.1) is the most common febrile exanthem in children younger than 3 years, occurring in about 30% of children. Onset of fever is abrupt and characteristically continuous, often as high as 40°C–41°C, and without a focus. Characteristically, the child becomes well and afebrile when the rash erupts.
- The patient's history should be searched for animal exposure, travel abroad, prior use of antibiotics, ingestion of raw milk, exposure to infection and consideration of ethnic group.
- Repeated physical examinations are more helpful in establishing a diagnosis than extensive investigations. A child with the initial diagnosis of PUO on presentation may often prove to have either a self-limiting benign disorder, such as viral infection (fever being the only sign of the disease), or a common disease with atypical presentation.
- Eye examination is essential and may suggest the diagnosis: bulbar conjunctivitis suggests Kawasaki's disease or leptospirosis; palpebral conjunctivitis may suggest TB, glandular fever or cat-scratch fever; petechial conjunctival haemorrhage suggests endocarditis;

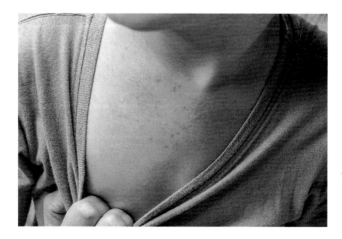

FIGURE 3.1   Exanthema subitum.

uveitis as an early clue for JRA or sarcoidosis; chorioretinitis suggests toxoplasmosis, syphilis, or CMV.

- Factitious fever, although rare, is an important cause of PUO (incidence: 1%–2% of causes of PUO). Measurement of temperature by a nurse attending to the procedure is essential to eliminate the rare possibility.
- Fever of neoplastic origin usually does not respond to antipyretics such as paracetamol, but it does respond to indomethacin or naproxen. Naproxen causes a prompt and complete lysis of neoplastic fever with sustained normal temperature (Naproxen test); Naproxen is therefore useful in the differential diagnosis between neoplastic and infectious fevers.

Red Flags

- Although viral infections account for the vast majority of causes of fever (90%–95%), children younger than 3 months of age, with immune deficiency (e.g. HIV or on chemotherapy), sickle-cell anaemia (SCA), cystic fibrosis (CF), asplenia, and with body temperature higher than 40°C should be considered as having bacterial infections until proven otherwise, and treatment with antibiotics should be commenced without waiting for laboratory results.
- Infants younger than 3 months of age and ill-appearing infants and children should be hospitalised, their urine and blood cultured, and they should receive IV ceftriaxone or cefotaxime. Those with fever higher than 39.0°C should be screened with blood WBC and CRP.
- Always remember that normal body temperature does not preclude serious bacterial infection.

FURTHER READING

El-Radhi AS. *Clinical Manual of Fever in Children*. New York, NY: Springer, 2018.

WEIGHT GAIN, EXCESSIVE (OBESITY)

Clinical Overview

Obesity is a common and serious problem in children. Its incidence has increased dramatically since 1970, and this rate is likely to continue. Overweight is defined as a body mass index (BMI) of greater than the 85th to less than the 95th centile, and obesity as greater than 95th for children. It is linked to adult obesity with the potential risk of increased mortality, cardiovascular disease, hypertension, diabetes, back pain, hyperlipidaemia, cholelithiasis and sleep apnoea. Obese children often do not eat more than their peers. Genetic factors and reduced energy output (long hours sitting in front of the TV and computer) are more important causal factors. Obesity is usually the result of increases in the number of fat cells (adipocytes) occurring during gestational months and the first year of life. Any early obesity may persist. Hormonal and endocrine causes of obesity are rare in clinical practise but often considered to be the reason by parents. There are currently no drugs available that can be recommended for use in children.

Possible Diagnoses

Infants	Children
Common	
Obese mother	Simple obesity
Infant of diabetic mother	Polycystic ovary syndrome (PCOS)
Post-term infants	Endocrine (e.g. Cushing's syndrome [CS])
Oedema (cardiac or renal)	Genetic syndromes (e.g. Turner's syndrome)
Drugs (e.g. steroids)	Drugs (e.g. steroids, pizotifen, anticonvulsants, antidepressants)
Rare	
Insulinoma	Cerebral gigantism (Sotos' syndrome)
Beckwith–Wiedemann syndrome	Oedema (renal or cardiac)
Cerebral gigantism (Sotos' syndrome)	Beckwith–Wiedemann syndrome
	Laurence–Moon–Biedl syndrome

Differential Diagnosis at a Glance

	Simple Obesity	PCOS	Endocrine (CS)	Genetic Syndrome	Drugs
Positive family history	Possible	No	No	Possible	No
More in females	No	Yes	No	Yes	No
Associated tall stature	Yes	No	No	No	Possible
Diagnostic tests available	No	Yes	Yes	Yes	Possible
Effective treatment available	No	Possible	Yes	No	Possible

Recommended Investigations

*** Urine: proteinuria in case of oedema caused by renal disease; free cortisol confirms CS
*** Thyroid function test (TFT): will confirm or exclude hypothyroidism
*** Urea and electrolytes (U&E) in blood: deranged in CS
*** Blood glucose for cases with non-insulin-dependent diabetes mellitus
*** Calcium and parathyroid hormone for cases with hypoparathyroidism

*** Serum cortisol levels will confirm CS
**   Bone age: normal in simple obesity, delayed
**   Pelvic ultrasound scan: will confirm ovarian cysts in PCOS; the adrenals for CS
**   Computed tomography (CT) scan or magnetic resonance imaging for suspected cases of CS

Top Tips

- Obesity due to a syndrome (e.g. Prader-Willi) or endocrine causes (e.g. hypothyroidism, CS) is rare. These children are differentiated from those with simple obesity by being short, with delayed bone age and delayed onset of secondary sexual characteristics. While fat distribution in simple obesity is diffuse, truncal obesity with thin legs is seen in CS.
- Striae in simple obesity are pink, occurring after rapid growth in adolescents, while these marks appear earlier in CS and are violaceous.
- A common reason for seeking medical help for child's obesity is parental concern about whether the 'child's glands' are normal. Obesity usually does not have 'glands' as an underlying cause.
- As BMI gives no indication of body fat distribution, waist circumference (midway between the tenth rib and top of the iliac crest) is a maker for central body fat accumulation and is more accurate than BMI.
- Much time is wasted in clinic by giving unwanted advice about food. The child with obesity is aware of that and often upset by frequently hearing that he or she is eating too much, and dietary restriction is notoriously unsuccessful in treating the condition.
- The main cause of childhood-onset obesity is not overeating, but genetics (usually confirmed by a detailed family history) and decreased energy output. The latter can be estimated indirectly by the total hours spent in front of the television and computer per day.

Red Flags

- Beware of the finding of supernumerary digit in an obese child: Laurence–Moon–Biedl syndrome (obesity, polydactyly, retinitis pigmentosa and progressive nephropathy) is likely.
- Do not miss another uncommon but important physical sign in an obese child: when the hand is clenched in a fist it may show short fourth and fifth knuckles – a sign seen in pseudohypoparathyroidism and in girls with Turner's syndrome.
- Record blood pressure in any child with obesity; it is elevated in those with CS and Turner's syndrome, and may also be elevated in simple obesity, sooner or later.
- Obesity may have child abuse (e.g. neglect) as an underlying cause. If such a case is suspected, prompt referral to appropriate service is essential.

FURTHER READING

Umer A, Kelley GA, Cottrell LE et al. Childhood obesity and adult cardiovascular disease risk factors: A systematic review with meta-analysis. *BMC Public Health* 2017;17:683.

4 FACE

ACUTE FACIAL PAIN

Clinical Overview

Facial pain, like any other pain, is an unpleasant sensory and emotional experience. The term is used to describe, on looking at the face, facial pain before a pain condition is diagnosed (pre-clinical pain). Facial trauma caused by an accident is excluded, as there is a clear cause for the pain. Facial pain has a long list of disorders including muscular-ligament inflammation (e.g. temporomandibular joint, salivary gland disease, sinusitis), dental (e.g. periodontal disease) and neurological causes (e.g. trigeminal neuralgia, cluster headache, post-herpetic neuralgia). Assessing facial pain and localising the source of the pain in children can be difficult, particularly in infants and young children. Nevertheless, diagnosis is usually possible by taking a good history and using pain assessment techniques classified as self-reporting, behavioural observation (such as facial expression, crying, forceful closure of the eyes) and physiologic measures (such as tachycardia, pupil dilatation).

Possible Diagnoses

Infants	Children
Common	
Otitis media	Headaches (e.g. migraine, particularly cluster pain)
Pharyngitis	Sinusitis
Facial osteomyelitis	Dental abscess
	Tumour (benign or malignant)
Rare	
Facial osteomyelitis	Temporomandibular joint dysfunction
	Glaucoma
	Persistent idiopathic facial pain
	Facial osteomyelitis (maxillary or mandibular)
	Herpes zoster (pre-rash appearance)
	Salivary gland disease
	Post-herpetic neuralgia (PHN)
	Post-traumatic trigeminal neuralgia
	Temporal arteritis
	Ramsay Hunt syndrome
	Trigeminal neuralgia (tic douloureux)

Differential Diagnosis at a Glance

	Headache	Sinusitis	Dental Abscess	Trigeminal Neuralgia	Facial Tumour
Associated swelling	No	No	Possible	No	Possible
Fever	No	Yes	Possible	No	No
Tenderness	Possible	Yes	Yes	No	Possible
Localised pain	No	Yes	Yes	Yes	Possible
Associated nausea/vomiting	Yes	Possible	No	Possible	No

Recommended Investigations

**   Full blood count (FBC): raised white blood cell (WBC) count in inflammatory conditions
**   C-reactive protein (CRP) and erythrocyte sedimentation rate (ESR): raised in infections, malignancy and temporal arteritis
**   X-ray of the face may show opacification of the sinus or mastoid area
**   Dental X-ray if a dental abscess is suspected
*** Computed tomography (CT)/magnetic resonance imaging (MRI) scan, which is more specific than an X-ray in diagnosing sinusitis or facial tumour
**   Sialography in suspected cases of parotid duct stone
**   Fine-needle biopsy for facial tumour
**   Tonometry: if glaucoma is suspected

Top Tips

- While the main site for neonatal facial osteomyelitis is the area of maxillary bone and pre-maxillary suture, the mandible is the usual location in older children. In both locations, children present with swelling, fever (rare in neonates), pain and redness of skin and oral mucosa.
- Adolescents and adults with sinusitis typically present with headaches, facial pain, tenderness and facial oedema, while symptoms of sinusitis in young children are persistence of upper respiratory tract infection, nasal discharge and cough that is typically worse when lying down.
- Trigeminal neuralgia is a sudden, severe, stabbing, usually unilateral pain of one or more branches of the fifth cranial nerve, which is often compressed. Tumour should be excluded.
- Idiopathic facial pain (previously called atypical facial pain) is a deep and poorly localised pain that is present daily for more than 2 hours a day over more than 3 months. There is no sensory loss. It is a diagnosis of exclusion.
- PHN is defined as pain persisting for more than 3 months after the onset of herpes zoster rash. Up to 50% of older people are estimated to develop PHN following shingles.
- Neuropathic pain (e.g. trigeminal neuralgia) is notoriously difficult to treat with opioids. Antidepressants (e.g. imipramine) and anticonvulsants (e.g. carbamazepine) are often effective.
- In managing pain, remember the stepwise approach, published by the World Health Organisation, to escalating therapy from weak analgesics (e.g. paracetamol or non-steroidal anti-inflammatory drugs) to strong ones (e.g. morphine).

Red Flags

- Although pressing over the area of the sinuses is the best direct method of examination, beware that the child might find any pressure on the face to be painful.
- Be aware that sinuses do not become potential infection sites in early childhood because they are not developed, so sinusitis should not be diagnosed in early childhood.
- Headaches may be the underlying disorder of facial pain. Remember that the three important causes are migraine (usually throbbing), tension headaches (usually 'pressing') and tumour with increased intracranial pressure producing throbbing, pressing or sharp pain.
- Neuropathic or persistent idiopathic facial pain is a challenge for dentists because the wrong dental diagnosis is often made, leading to the wrong treatment.

FURTHER READING

Zakrzewski JM. Facial pain: Neurological and non-neurological. *J Neurol Neurosurg Psychiatry* 2002;72(Suppl 2): 27–32.

FACIAL RASH

Clinical Overview

A child's skin is more reactive than an adult's. For example, vesiculo-bullous eruptions are more common in children, and many systemic diseases present with cutaneous manifestations. In addition, the appearance of macules or patches does not commonly remain static, and acute eruption can change rapidly to become elevated (maculopapular) or blistering (maculovesicular). Facial rash in this section is classified according to a simple practical approach based on the morphological appearance of the rash:

- Macule (<1 cm) and patch (>1 cm): defined as alteration of skin colour but no elevation is felt
- Papule (<1 cm), nodule (>1 cm) and tumour (>nodule)
- Vesicle (1 cm) and bulla (>1 cm): defined as fluid-filled, raised lesions
- Purpura, extravasation of blood, occurs with petechiae (pin-point) or ecchymoses (patches)
- Eruptions can be a mixture of lesions such as maculopapular, papulo-vesicular or vesiculo-bullous
- Vascular and pigmented birthmarks are not included in this section; see Chapter 14.

Possible Diagnoses

Infants	Children
Common	
Papulo-vesicular (e.g. atopic dermatitis)	Macules/patches (e.g. viral infections, allergy)
Macules or patches (e.g. viral infectious diseases)	Papules (e.g. insect bites, scabies)
Patch (salmon patch)	Papulo-vesicular (e.g. atopic dermatitis)
Papulo-pustular (e.g. erythema toxicum)	Vesiculo-pustular (e.g. non-bullous impetigo)
Papules (e.g. seborrhoeic dermatitis [SD])	Purpuric (e.g. meningococcaemia)
Rare	
Bullae (e.g. bullous impetigo)	Bullae (epidermolysis bullosa, bullous impetigo)
Vesiculo-bullous (e.g. herpes infections)	Nodular (e.g. angio-fibroma in tuberous sclerosis)
	Papulo-pustulo-nodular (e.g. acne)
	Vesiculo-bullous (e.g. herpes infections)
	Papule-plagues (e.g. lichen planus)
	Patch, periorbital, violaceous (dermatomyositis)
	Papulo-squamous (e.g. psoriasis, pityriasis rosea)
	Vesicles, linear (poison ivy, contact dermatitis)

Differential Diagnosis at a Glance

	Macules	Papules	Papulo-Vesicular	Vesico-Pustular	Purpuric
Itchy	Possible	Yes	Yes	Possible	No
Associated fever	Yes	No	No	No	Yes
Rash elsewhere	Yes	No	No	No	Yes
Ill-looking	Possible	No	No	No	Yes
Respond to local treatment	No	Yes	Yes	Yes	No

Recommended Investigations

** FBC: leukopenia in some viral diseases, e.g. measles, leukocytosis (e.g. HHV-6)
** CRP: high in bacterial diseases, e.g. meningococcal disease
*** BC for suspected cases of meningococcaemia
** Auto-antibodies, e.g. ANA, double-stranded DNA in systemic lupus erythematosus
*** Muscle enzymes (e.g. creatine phosphokinase)
*** MRI and muscle biopsy for dermatomyositis

Top Tips

- In contrast to atopic dermatitis (AD), SD is usually present within the first month of life, disappears when the child is aged 1–2 years, and is usually non-pruritic.
- Among those rashes causing intense pruritis are urticaria, AD and lichen planus.
- Pruritis from any cause is always worse at night. The warmth of bedclothes causes vasodilatation in the skin, which worsens the itching. Ask parents how well their child sleeps at night.
- AD should be diagnosed with strict criteria for both major factors (e.g. family or personal history of atopy, typical facial or extensor lesions) and minor (elevated IgE, xerosis, susceptibility for infection).
- Urticaria (mostly caused by drugs, food or viruses) is often confused with erythema multiforme. The latter produces typical iris or target lesions, and mucosal involvement is common.
- Although drugs can cause a variety of cutaneous morphologies, the most common drug-induced rashes are urticaria, erythema multiforme and maculopapular eruptions.
- Juvenile dermatomyositis (JDM) is now part of inflammatory idiopathic myopathies. JDM is characterised by proximal muscle weakness, facial heliotrope rash and Gottron's papules.

Red Flags

- Remember to examine the buccal mucosa in any child presenting with a rash. Examples include reticulate, white plaques in lichen planus and vesiculo-bullous lesions in erythema multiforme.
- In children with pruritic skin eruption, treating the pruritis is more important than the rash.
- Although purpura is the most common rash of meningococcal disease, other rashes include maculopapular, pustular and bullous lesions.
- Be aware that rash due to sunburn may occur in cloudy weather without sun exposure.
- Children with AD are at risk of a serious complication with herpes simplex virus – eczema herpeticum – which can be fatal. Intravenous acyclovir is the mainstay of treatment.
- Be aware that in children with cold urticaria, pruritic painful rash appears on exposure to cold on exposed parts of the body. Swimming in cold water is dangerous and can be fatal.

FURTHER READING

Van Dijkhuizen EHP, De Iorio M, Wedderburn LR et al. Clinical signs and symptoms in a joint model of four disease activity parameters in juvenile dermatomyositis: A prospective, longitudinal, multicenter cohort study. *Arthritis Res Ther* 2018;20:180.

FACIAL SWELLING

Clinical Overview

Facial swelling is a common clinical paediatric problem. The term refers to an enlargement of any area of the face, including the eyes, nose, mouth, forehead, cheeks and chin. Swelling is usually caused by an abnormal buildup of fluid in the face – oedema – which is the most common cause of facial swelling. Oedema is either generalised – caused by systemic diseases such as nephrotic syndrome (NS), glomerulonephritis, congestive cardiac failure (CCF), acute and chronic renal failure (ARF and CRF) or hypoproteinaemia – or localised – caused by allergy such as angioneurotic oedema or bee sting. Genuine oedema needs to be differentiated from 'puffy face', which is often found in association with obesity, hypothyroidism and Cushing's syndrome. Facial masses are the second most common causes of facial swelling.

Possible Diagnoses

Infants	Children
Common	
Oedema (acute illness, excess IV fluid)	Dental abscess
Electrolyte imbalance (e.g. prematurity)	Haemangioma
ARF	Salivary gland diseases (mumps, duct stone < tumour)
CCF	Allergy (angioneurotic oedema, bee sting)
Lymphoedema	Generalised oedema (e.g. NS)
Rare	
Haemangioma, teratoma	Infections (e.g. sinusitis, HIV, trichinosis)
Parotid swelling (e.g. neonatal parotitis)	Midline dermoid cyst
	Lymphoedema, lymphangioma
	Hereditary angioedema (HAE)
	Subcutaneous emphysema
	Tuberculosis, sarcoidosis
	Renal failure
	Superior vena cava obstruction
	Tumour (e.g. rhabdomyosarcoma, Ewing's sarcoma)
	Metastatic neuroblastoma

Differential Diagnosis at a Glance

	Dental Abscess	Haemangioma	Salivary Gland Diseases	Allergy	Generalised
Acute onset	Possible	No	Possible	Yes	Yes
Associated pain	Yes	No	Possible	No	No
Unilateral	Yes	Yes	Yes	No	No
Associated itch	No	No	No	Yes	No
Swelling elsewhere	No	No	No	Yes	Yes

Recommended Investigations

*** Urine for protein in NS or glomerulonephritis, and for free cortisol for Cushing's syndrome

*** Blood for serum urea and electrolytes, albumin and triglyceride in suspected NS

**   Blood for RAST (or skin prick test) for allergy; C1 esterase for hereditary angioedema
***   Blood for dexamethasone suppression test for Cushing's syndrome
***   Chest X-ray, electrocardiogram and echocardiography to diagnose the cause of CCF
**   Ultrasound scan is useful for suspected facial tumours such as a parotid tumour
***   CT scan or MRI for sinusitis and underlying tumours
***   Sialography and/or sialendoscopy to demonstrate salivary duct stone

Top Tips

- A premature infant is at high risk of developing generalised oedema, including facial oedema, because of low glomerular infiltration rate and an inability to handle water and solute loads.
- Dental abscess is due to bacterial infection of the dental pulp or the gum (periodontal abscess).
- Sinusitis can be easily diagnosed clinically: children have fever (50%–60%), mid-face pressure tenderness and/or pain, nasal secretion and obstruction and hyposmia.
- Angio-oedema (or angioneurotic oedema) is similar to urticaria, except it affects the deeper layers of subcutaneous and mucous tissues. Its intense pruritis and redness differentiate it from generalised oedema caused, for example, by hypoproteinaemia.
- There are 700–1,000 salivary glands in the oropharynx, in three major areas (parotid, submandibular, sublingual). Adults produce *c*. 1.5 L of saliva daily, >70% from the sub-mandibular gland.
- Recurrent parotitis presents as acute swelling of the affected gland due to either congenital causes (e.g. dilatation of the duct causing saliva stasis) or a stone obstructing the saliva's passage.
- Lymphoedema – non-pitting oedema of the face – is either congenital (e.g. Milroy's disease, Turner's syndrome in girls, Noonan's syndrome in boys) or acquired following removal of lymph nodes for biopsy or radiation therapy for cancer; rarely it is caused by filariasis infection.

Red Flags

- Remember that an acute dental abscess may be painless and present as fever, chills or pyrexia of unknown origin (PUO). Dental abscess needs to be excluded in any case of PUO.
- Rapidly progressive facial swelling may suggest a malignant tumour such as rhabdomyosarcoma, while slowly progressive facial swelling is often caused by less serious conditions such as fibrous dysplasia, haemangioma or neurofibroma.
- Facial swelling may be caused by superior vena cava obstruction, which manifests as swollen face especially around the eyes, distended neck and prominent chest veins.
- Beware that HIV may initially present as painful or painless parotid swelling.
- Children with episodic hereditary angioedema are at risk of potentially fatal laryngeal swelling. It is essential that all family members, including infants, are investigated.
- If a child presents with swelling of the glabella area (area between the eyebrows), then encephalocele, nasal glioma or midline or nasal dermoid cyst should be excluded. Encephaloceles have an intracranial connection; 25% of cases of dermoid cyst have intracranial connection.
- Intranasal encephalocele can be seen hanging in the nasal cavity, and can be mistaken as a polyp. Its removal causes serious complications such as CSF liquorrhoea and/or meningitis.

FURTHER READING

Ivo H, Zenk J. Salivary gland diseases in children. *GMS Curr Top Otorhinolaryngol Head Neck Surg* 2014;13:Doc06.

FACIAL WEAKNESS

Clinical Overview

Facial weakness may be congenital or acquired, idiopathic or caused by infection, inflammation, trauma, tumour or a vascular event. The most common cause of congenital facial weakness is trauma during delivery. The most common cause of acquired facial weakness is Bell's palsy, which is an idiopathic, isolated lower motor-neuron lesion of the seventh nerve characterised by sudden onset weakness. As a rule, children with facial weakness have better prognosis than adults. Facial weakness should be differentiated from facial asymmetry, which may result from underdevelopment of the muscle controlling the lip, excessive moulding of the cranium, or face presentation during delivery, or in older children with hemihypertrophy.

Possible Diagnoses

Infants	Children
Common	
Birth injury (e.g. forceps delivery)	Bell's palsy
Congenital myasthenia	Infection (e.g. Lyme disease, herpes zoster)
Congenital myopathies (e.g. nemaline)	Myopathies (myotonic dystrophy)
Möbius syndrome	
Agenesis of depressor angularis oris muscle	Myasthenia gravis
Rare	
Transient myasthenia gravis	Agenesis of the depressor angularis oris muscle
Coloboma, heart defect, atresia rate of the choanae, retarded growth, genital hypoplasia and ear anomaly (CHARGE) association	CHARGE association
Bell's palsy	Chronic ataxic neuropathy with ophthalmoplegia, M-protein, agglutination and disialosyl antibodies (CANOMAD)
	Guillain–Barré syndrome
Goldenhar's syndrome	Ramsay Hunt syndrome
	Neuro-sarcoidosis
	Poland's syndrome
	Hypertension
	Möbius syndrome

Differential Diagnosis at a Glance

	Bell's Palsy	Infection	Myopathy	Möbius Syndrome	Myasthenia
Congenital	No	No	Possible	Yes	Possible
Facial weakness only	Yes	Possible	No	No	No
Unilateral	Yes	Possible	No	No	No
Lower motor	Yes	Yes	Yes	No	Yes
Sudden onset	Yes	Possible	No	No	No

Recommended Investigations

*** Anti-acetylcholine and anti-nuclear antibodies for myasthenia

*** Edrophonium test (0.2 mg/kg IV) in myasthenia

*** Electromyogram: more specifically diagnostic than a muscle biopsy in myasthenia gravis
*** Neuroimaging: for cases not recovering
** Nerve conduction studies
* Muscle biopsy has limited value in myasthenia

Top Tips

- Unilateral facial weakness due to forceps delivery has an almost 100% recovery rate, while the recovery rate of older children with the acquired form of Bell's palsy is 80%–90%.
- Bell's palsy affects the taste of two-thirds of the anterior tongue and salivary and lacrimal glands. Early effects include difficulty in eating, difficulty in speech and corneal dryness. Later symptoms include pain around the ear, altered taste, involuntary facial spasm and impaired lacrimation.
- Möbius syndrome is congenital hypoplasia of the motor nuclei of III, IV and V, in addition to VII.
- Conditions often mistaken as facial weakness include hemihypertrophy (congenital overgrowth often involving the size or length of extremities, but it may involve the face) and Goldenhar's syndrome (oculo-auriculo-vertebral with hypoplastic malar and maxilla on one side and sensory neural deafness) due to a defect of the first two branchial arches.
- CANOMAD syndrome is a rare immune-mediated demyelinating polyneuropathy.

Red Flags

- Facial palsy in neonates is not apparent until crying, when the facial asymmetry becomes clear.
- Gradual onset of facial weakness over 2–3 weeks may suggest a neoplastic cause.
- Patients with facial weakness suffer from impaired verbal communication and social interaction, leading to emotional stress and social isolation. Treatment is urgent and essential.
- In Lyme disease, caused by the spirochete *Borrelia burgdorferi*, facial nerve palsy may be the initial or the only manifestation of the disease.
- Patients with facial palsy are not able to close the eye on the affected side, leading to keratitis and corneal ulceration. Protection of the cornea with eye drops is of paramount importance.
- Agenesis of depressor angularis oris muscle – also termed *asymmetric facial crying* or *congenital unilateral lower lip palsy* (CULLP) – is a congenital defect due to underdevelopment of the muscle controlling the lip. It is often mistaken as facial palsy; the lesion is permanent.
- An uncommon cause of facial weakness is acoustic neuroma, occurring either as a sporadic form or in association with neurofibromatosis type 2. Children present with hearing loss (the most common symptom, in 95%), vertigo and tinnitus.

FURTHER READING

Ciorba A, Corazzi V, Con V et al. Facial nerve paralysis in children. *World J Clin Cases* 2015;3(12):973–979.

5 NECK

Clinical Overview

Pathologies in the larynx in children are caused by four main groups: acute infection, airway stenosis, tumours and foreign body. The term *dysphonia* includes any impairment of the voice or alteration in the sound of the voice. Hoarseness subsequent to an acute upper airway obstruction (causing croup) in association with a viral upper respiratory tract infection (URTI) is by far the most common presentation in children. Croup is characterised by abrupt onset at night, with barking cough, inspiratory stridor and respiratory distress. Mild obstruction usually causes transient symptoms (hoarseness and stridor). More severe degrees of obstruction cause more persistent symptoms of stridor and hoarseness, nasal flaring and subcostal and intercostal recession. Recovery within a few days is usually the rule. On rare occasions such an obstruction is caused by more serious underlying causes, such as *Staphylococcal aureus* (causing bacterial tracheitis) and *Haemophilus influenzae* type b (causing epiglottitis). The obstruction is more serious in infants and young children than in older children because of the smaller airway and the more likely obstruction. Persistent hoarseness usually suggests cord paralysis or tumours. In this section, abnormal or unusual voices are included.

Possible Diagnoses

Infants	Children
Common	
Trauma to vocal cords	Laryngotracheobronchitis (croup)
Excessive crying	Spasmodic croup
Prolonged ventilation (vocal nodule)	Angioedema
Central nervous system disease (Chiari malformation)	Overuse of the voice (excessive crying)
Viral laryngotracheobronchitis	Vocal cord abnormality (e.g. haemangioma)
Rare	
Benign tumour (haemangioma)	Corticosteroid inhalation therapy
Cri-du-chat syndrome (5p-deletion)	Bacterial tracheitis (staphylococcal infection)
	Epiglottitis
	Gastro-oesophageal (GO) reflux
	Juvenile recurring papillomatosis
	Infectious mononucleosis
	Aspiration of foreign body
	Tumour (e.g. papilloma, rhabdomyosarcoma)
	Hypothyroidism
	Vocal cord paralysis (postoperative)
	Wegener's disease
	Rheumatoid arthritis
	Systemic lupus erythematosus

(Continued)

(Continued)

Infants	Children
	Measles croup
	Chemotherapy toxicity (e.g. vincristine, cisplatin)
	Retropharyngeal or peritonsillar abscess
	Laryngeal abscess
	Hypocalcaemic tetany
	Laryngeal sarcoidosis
	Amyloidosis

Differential Diagnosis at a Glance

	Viral Croup	Spasmodic Croup	Angioedema	Overuse of Voice	Vocal Cord Abnormality
Fever	Possible	No	No	No	No
Preceded by URTI	Yes	No	No	No	No
Onset at night	Yes	Yes	No	No	No
Skin eruption	No	No	Yes	No	No
Stridor	Yes	Yes	Possible	Possible	Yes

Recommended Investigations

Most cases of acute hoarseness and stridor do not need any investigation.

** Thyroid function tests to exclude hypothyroidism
** Serum calcium to confirm hypocalcaemia
** Blood culture indicated for suspected cases of epiglottitis
*** Direct laryngoscopy to diagnose laryngeal haemangiomas and paralysis of the vocal cord
** Chest X-ray may diagnose vascular ring or aspiration
** Computed tomography scan or magnetic resonance imaging of the head to diagnose Chiari malformation

Top Tips

- Laryngeal injury may occur subsequent to birth trauma, resulting in unilateral vocal cord paralysis producing hoarseness and stridor. In addition, bilateral paralysis causes dyspnoea.
- GO reflux is an important cause of laryngospasm or vocal cord dysfunction. Presentation is usually with cough, vomiting and feeding problems, in addition to hoarseness.
- Differentiating viral croup from spasmodic croup is easy: the latter is not associated with fever, has no antecedent URTI, and symptoms are more transient compared to viral croup.
- The prognosis of viral and spasmodic croup is excellent. About 1%–2% of children with laryngotracheobronchitis have severe symptoms requiring intensive care and intubation.
- Inhaled corticosteroids are the most effective medication for asthma control. Adverse effects include hoarseness, candidiasis, cough reflex and pharyngitis. Effect on the vocal cords is due to 'steroid myopathy' causing deformity and bowing of the vocal muscles.
- Juvenile recurring papillomatosis usually occurs between the ages of 2 and 4 years and is a major cause of hoarseness. The infection is caused by peri-partum transmission of human papillomavirus (HPV). Type HPV-11 may lead to obstruction of the respiratory tract, requiring tracheostomy.

Red Flags

- Bilateral vocal cord paralysis may lead to recurrent pneumonia caused by recurrent aspiration.
- In contrast to lower respiratory tract obstruction, children with croup do not usually have hypoxia (normal oxygen saturation); if hypoxia is detected, prompt treatment is needed.
- Symptoms of laryngotracheobronchitis do not usually continue for more than a few days. Persistent hoarseness requires laryngoscopy to detect the cause.
- A child with 'croup' who rapidly becomes unwell with sternal retraction and decreased level of consciousness, with or without fever, either has extension of the croup into the respiratory tract pending respiratory failure (bacterial tracheitis) or has bacterial epiglottitis.
- A young child (6 months–2 years) with sudden choking and coughing, with or without stridor or hoarseness, should be suspected of foreign-body aspiration.
- As part of anaphylaxis and severe allergic reaction, sudden onset of angioedema of the subglottic areas may occur. Adrenaline injection is life-saving.
- Papilloma is the most common tumour of the larynx. Although usually benign and often regressing at the time of puberty, it can extend into the lower airways and lungs, causing a serious disease.

FURTHER READING

McAllister A, Sjölander P. Children's voice and voice disorders. *Semin Speech Lang* 2013;34:71–79.
Reiter R, Hoffmann TK, Pickhard A et al. The hypothesis of apraxia of speech in children with autism spectrum disorder. *J Autism Dev Disord* 2011;41(4):405–426.

NECK LUMPS (LYMPHADENOPATHY)

Clinical Overview

Lumps in the neck are common and are usually benign in children. Of the many lumps found in the neck, cervical lymphadenopathy is the most common physical finding. It usually results from viral infection leaving behind small (<1 cm), non-tender mobile lymph nodes, which are considered normal in children. Lymph nodes are considered enlarged when their diameter exceeds 1 cm for cervical and axillary lymph nodes and 1.5 cm for inguinal lymph nodes. Cervical lymph nodes drain lymph from the head and neck areas; submental and submandibular lymph nodes drain from the buccal mucosa, cheek and nose; supraclavicular lymph nodes drain from right-sided thorax and left-sided abdomen; axillary drain from the ipsilateral arm, breast and neck; and inguinal lymph nodes drain from the ipsilateral leg and buttocks. About one-third of neonates have palpable lymph nodes, usually smaller than 1 cm in diameter. They are commonly present in the inguinal area due to infection of the nappy area. Generalised lymphadenopathy indicates involvement of enlarged lymph nodes in more than two node regions. Pathological lymphadenopathy is defined by abnormally large lymph nodes with tenderness, matted together or fixed to the skin or underlying structures, or localised in the supraclavicular area.

Possible Diagnoses

Infants	Children
Common	
Lymphadenopathy	Reactive lymphadenitis due to local infection
Goiter	Systemic infection (e.g. Kawasaki disease, mononucleosis)
Sternomastoid tumour	Goiter
Dermoid cyst	Malignancy (e.g. lymphoma, rhabdomyosarcoma)
Thyroglossal cyst	Thyroglossal cyst
Rare	
Cystic hygroma	Juvenile idiopathic arthritis (JIA)
Branchial cyst	Tuberculosis (TB) lymphadenitis
	Cat-scratch fever
	Systemic lupus erythematosus (SLE)
	Kaposi's sarcoma, teratoma
	Lipoma, dermoid cyst
	Drugs (INH, phenytoin)

Differential Diagnosis at a Glance

	Reactive Lymphadenitis	Systemic Disease	Goiter	Lymphoma	Thyroglossal Cyst
Tender	Possible	Possible	No	No	No
Generalised	Possible	Yes	No	Possible	No
Moves with swallowing	No	No	No	No	Yes
Midline	No	No	Yes	No	Yes
Fixed to skin	No	No	No	Yes	No

Recommended Investigations

*** Chest X-ray: first-line investigation and helpful in case of TB or lymphoma
**   Ultrasound of the neck is useful for any lump
*** Full blood count (FBC): leukocytosis favours bacterial infection; atypical lymphocytes for mononucleosis

** Liver function tests: abnormal in Epstein–Barr virus (EBV) or cytomegalovirus (CMV)
** EBV serological panel test or IgG for EBV
*** Tuberculin skin test for suspected TB adenitis
** Serum antibody studies for EBV, CMV, HIV, or bartonella (cat-scratch fever)
*** Needle aspiration for a Gram stain and culture in suspected malignancy

Top Tips

- Lymph nodes act as a filter between lymphatic and haematological circulations. They contain immunological cells including macrophages, B cells and T cells.
- The most common neck lump is reactive lymphadenopathy, usually caused by a viral infection. The condition is benign, but the lymph nodes may remain as harmless palpable lumps for months or years. Parents usually fear the possibility of cancer; it is important to reassure them.
- Generalised lymphadenopathy suggests either systemic infection (e.g. AIDS, mononucleosis, toxoplasmosis), autoimmune disease (e.g. JIA) or malignancy (e.g. leukaemia).
- A thyroglossal cyst, which develops from the remnant thyroglossal duct, is painless but becomes enlarged and tender if infected. The pathognomonic sign is its vertical movement on swallowing and tongue protrusion. These cysts are the second most common neck masses after lymph nodes.
- The usual branchial cyst looks like an insignificant papule on the side of the neck, off centre (in contrast to thyroglossal cyst). Tracing out its tract in surgical removal may be quite difficult.
- The most common acquired goiter in children is Hashimoto's thyroiditis, presenting with normal thyroid function or hypothyroidism.
- JIA often presents with generalised lymphadenopathy, seen mostly in systemic form (Still's disease) in association with fever, rash and hepatosplenomegaly.

Red Flags

- Be aware that some lymph nodes are present in virtually any child; the total absence of palpable lymph nodes suggests the possibility of immune deficiency such as agammaglobulinaemia.
- Cervical lymphadenopathy is often among the initial presentations in HIV-infected patients. Look for oral candida or gingivitis to support the diagnosis.
- Painless generalised lymphadenopathy may precede the other symptoms of SLE by months or years. Screening for SLE may clinch the diagnosis.
- Be very cautious in undertaking needle aspiration for TB lymphadenitis as there is a real risk of fistula.
- Urgent referral is indicated if the lymph nodes are matted or fixed, >2 cm in diameter, non-tender, less mobile or associated with persistent or unexplained fever, night sweat, or anorexia or weight loss. Fine-needle aspiration has a high specificity and is less invasive, cheaper and quicker.
- Kawasaki disease may present with fever and cervical lymphadenopathy only. Bacterial lymphadenitis is often diagnosed, thus delaying diagnosis, and treatment can lead to serious cardiac complications.
- A thyroglossal cyst should never be excised unless the possibility of thyroid tissue is excluded.
- Thyroid nodules are uncommon in children compared to adults, but are often malignant in up to 25%.

FURTHER READING

Lang S, Kansy B. Cervical lymph node diseases in children. *GMC Curr Top Otorhinolaryngol Head Neck Surg* 2014;13:Doc08.

SORE THROAT AND MOUTH

Clinical Overview

Sore throat and sore mouth are common in children. According to the World Health Organisation, approximately 600 million new cases of acute tonsillo-pharyngitis caused by group A streptococci (GAS) occur annually in children worldwide. Of these, 15.6 million develop rheumatic heart disease, with 233,000 deaths each year, mostly in developing countries. The most common cause in young children is a viral URTI, including pharyngitis. An infection rate of 6–8 infections a year is considered a normal range. Higher incidence is found in infants and children who attend nursery and whose siblings attend nursery or school. Acute pharyngitis refers to the pharynx as the principal site of the inflammatory process. Viruses (e.g. adenoviruses, EBV) and bacteria (most commonly GAS) have overlapping symptoms and signs, and clinically they are often indistinguishable from each other. This infection is uncommon in children younger than 1 year of age, peaks at the age of 4–7 years and continues throughout later childhood.

Possible Diagnoses

Infants	Children
Common	
Viral URTI	Viral tonsillo-pharyngitis (with URTI)
With exanthem (measles, varicella)	Bacterial tonsillitis
Herpetic gingivostomatitis	Glandular fever (GF)
Croup	Herpetic gingivostomatitis
Bacterial tonsillo-pharyngitis	With exanthem (e.g. measles, varicella)
Rare	
Oropharyngeal thrush	Kawasaki disease
Kawasaki disease	Scarlet fever
Herpangina	Herpangina
Diphtheria	Immunodeficiency (e.g. HIV infection)
	Leukopenia/neutropenia
	Epiglottitis
	Retropharyngeal abscess
	Peritonsillar abscess
	Psychogenic
	Diphtheria
	Oropharyngeal thrush
	Aphthous ulceration

Differential Diagnosis at a Glance

	Viral Tonsillo-Pharyngitis	Bacterial Tonsillo-Pharyngitis	Glandular Fever	Herpetic Stomatitis	With Exanthem
Gingival lesions	No	No	No	Yes	Possible
Lymphadenopathy	Possible	Yes	Yes	Possible	Possible
Response to antibiotics	No	Yes	No	No	No
Associated URTI	Yes	No	No	No	Yes
Exudate on tonsils	Yes	Yes	Yes	No	No

Recommended Investigations

*** FBC may show leukocytosis in bacterial infection or lymphocytosis in GF

** Throat swab to culture GAS may be useful

** An antistreptolysin (ASO)-titre with fourfold increase in 1–2 weeks is diagnostic for streptococcal infection

*** EBV serological panel is useful to diagnose glandular fever; IgM for EBV is positive in almost 100%

Top Tips

- The main reasons for antibiotic therapy of bacterial pharyngitis are not only to treat the symptoms, but also to prevent complications (e.g. peritonsillar abscess, rheumatic fever and glomerulonephritis).
- The vast majority of cases of tonsillo-pharyngitis are caused by viral infections in association with an URTI; antibiotics therefore are not indicated for the majority of cases.
- Streptococci colonisation occurs in 10%–20% of normal school-aged children, as shown by positive swab culture. They are not at risk of developing rheumatic fever or glomerulonephritis. Antibiotics are not helpful for clearing GAS.
- In contrast to herpetic stomatitis caused by herpes virus, which has lesions on the gingiva, in herpangina (caused by coxsackievirus), there are discrete punctate vesicles surrounded by erythematous rings on the soft palate, anterior pillars and uvula.
- Tonsillectomy or partial tonsillectomy (tonsillotomy) is recommended for recurrent tonsillitis (equal to or more than the episodes in the preceding year), peritonsillar abscess, and PFAPA (periodic fever, aphthous stomatitis, pharyngitis and cervical adenitis).

Red Flags

- Many systemic diseases (e.g. Crohn's disease, agranulocytosis) manifest in the oral cavity as mucosal changes, which present clinically as sore throat. Look for an underlying disease.
- In suspected epiglottitis (toxic-looking, high fever, muffled voice), the throat should not be inspected. The child is to be transported to accident and emergency in consultation with ear, nose and throat (ENT) and anaesthesia.
- In mononucleosis, antibiotics (amoxicillin) should not be administered, to prevent skin eruption. Serious complications are rare but should be considered, including airway obstruction secondary to oropharyngeal inflammation, spontaneous splenic rupture and Hodgkin's lymphoma.
- Children with obstructive sleep apnoea (OSA), caused by adenotonsillar hypertrophy, are at risk of growth retardation and cardiovascular and neuro-behavioural complications. Referral to ENT with consideration of tonsillectomy is strongly indicated.
- If there is unexplained oropharyngeal candida infection, consider immunosuppression (HIV).
- A torn frenum detected at oral examination is widely regarded as pathognomonic of child abuse. Parents/carers usually offer an inadequate explanation for the injury.
- Symptoms of laryngotracheobronchitis do not usually continue for more than a few days. Persistent hoarseness requires laryngoscopy to detect the cause.

- A child with 'croup' who rapidly becomes unwell with high fever either has developed extension of the infection into the respiratory tract (bacterial tracheitis) as a complication of the viral croup or has bacterial epiglottitis.
- A young child (6 months–2 years) with sudden choking, coughing, with or without stridor or hoarseness, should be suspected of having foreign-body aspiration.
- As part of anaphylaxis and a severe allergic reaction, sudden onset of angioedema of the subglottic areas may occur. Epinephrine injection is life-saving.
- Papilloma is the most common tumour of the larynx. Although usually benign and often regressing at the time of puberty, it can extend into the lower airways and lungs, causing serious disease.

FURTHER READING

Carapetis JR, Steer AC, Mulholland EK et al. The global burden of group A streptococcal diseases. *Lancet Infect Dis* 2005;5(11):685–694.

STIFF NECK

Clinical Overview

This symptom is extremely important because of the possibility of meningitis and other serious bacterial infections such as pneumonia. It is a common complaint in paediatrics for both emergency and primary care services. The term refers to abnormal position of the neck or restricted range of movement, usually associated with pain during passive and active movement. Of the many causes of stiff neck, the two main and important causes are meningitis and torticollis (wry neck), which is characterised by tilting and rotation of the head to one side, with restricted rotation towards the opposite side. In infants, it is usually caused by a shortening sternomastoid muscle after the formation of swelling (called sternomastoid tumour); another possible cause is cervical spine abnormality. Meningism is the other important cause and always requires emergency evaluation. It is characterised by the presence of signs of neck stiffness in flexion position. The most common cause of meningism is meningeal irritation (meningitis or cerebral haemorrhage). In contrast to torticollis, a child with meningism is usually ill-looking with fever. Cerebrospinal fluid examination is usually required to exclude meningitis.

Possible Diagnoses

Infants	Children
Common	
Muscular torticollis (sternomastoid tumour, cerebral palsy)	Meningitis, meningococcal disease
Sandifer syndrome (GO reflux)	Pneumonia (e.g. upper lobe pneumonia)
Congenital abnormalities of cervical spine	Cervical lymphadenitis
Klippel–Feil syndrome	Acute torticollis (cervical muscle trauma)
Meningitis	Neck injury (whiplash injury)
	Infectious mononucleosis
Rare	
Muscular cervical injury	Visual defects (nystagmus, superior oblique paresis)
Pterygium colli	Dystonia
	Hysteria
	Vertebral anomalies (e.g. Klippel–Feil malformation)
	Rheumatoid arthritis
	Lyme disease (LD)
	Polymyalgia rheumatica
	Chiari malformation
	Posterior fossa brain tumour
	Intracranial haemorrhage
	Retropharyngeal abscess
	Spasmus nutans

Differential Diagnosis at a Glance

	Meningitis	Pneumonia	Cervical Lymphadenitis	Acute Torticollis	Cervical Injury
Toxic appearance	Yes	Yes	No	No	Possible
High fever	Yes	Yes	Possible	No	No
Positive meningeal signs	Yes	No	No	No	No
Vomiting/headaches	Yes	Possible	No	Possible	No
History of trauma	No	No	No	Possible	Yes

Recommended Investigations

** FBC: leukocytosis suggests bacterial infection in meningitis and pneumonia

*** Lumbar puncture to exclude meningitis; for cases with aseptic meningitis, enterovirus polymerase chain reaction should be tested for

** In the presence of pulmonary symptoms, a chest X-ray is required to diagnose pneumonia

** Cervical X-ray to diagnose spinal abnormalities such as fusion of the vertebrae

** Renal ultrasound scan to diagnose renal malformation (e.g. Klippel–Feil syndrome)

Top Tips

- Torticollis from sternomastoid tumor is initially minimal. At 10–20 days, a mass is frequently felt in the muscle that gradually disappears; the fibrous tissue contracts, causing limited head motion.
- Mild neck stiffness following sleep may result from sleeping in an awkward position. Gentle active rotation and flexion are usually achievable.
- Children with torticollis and dystonic drug reaction look remarkably well despite the stiff neck, in contrast to those with meningitis or pneumonia.
- A child with Klippel–Feil malformation (short neck, fusion of the cervical vertebrae) has a high rate of renal malformations (40%).
- Any child with meningism should be considered as a case of meningitis until it is proved otherwise.
- Most cases of congenital torticollis are due to sternomastoid tumour, which is usually palpable on the sternomastoid muscle. The torticollis responds to physiotherapy. Those infants with no history of birth trauma and no palpable mass should have anterio-posterior and lateral spine X-rays to exclude structural abnormalities before starting physiotherapy.
- In any with stiff neck, it is important to assess the immunization status of the child.

Red Flags

- In infants, early presentations of meningitis can be subtle and non-specific, often with irritability without fever. Bulging fontanelle or signs of meningeal irritation are late signs of meningitis.
- In older children, the classical signs of meningitis (fever, headache, vomiting, neck stiffness) may not occur; rather they may present with virus-like illness and a mixture of leg pain, drowsiness, confusion, neck pain, seizure and behavioural changes. Within a few hours it can rapidly progress to septic shock, hypotension, disseminated intravascular coagulation and death. Vigilance and a high degree of suspicion are required.
- Skin of a child with meningism should be carefully searched for any rash or petechiae of meningococcal disease.
- Even if pneumonia is diagnosed, a child with meningism requires LP to exclude meningitis.
- Drug history is essential to confirm a rare case of dystonic drug reaction (oculogyric crisis).
- Although acquired torticollis is mostly due to minor cervical muscle trauma or an URTI, careful evaluation is essential to exclude serious conditions such as a brain tumour or vertebral infection.

FURTHER READING

Dorsett M, Liang SY. Diagnosis and treatment of central nervous system infections in the emergency department. *Emerg Med Clin North Am* 2016;34(4):917–942.

STRIDOR

Clinical Overview

There are four main groups of pathologies in the larynx in children: acute infection, airway stenosis, tumours and foreign body. Stridor is a harsh inspiratory sound caused by extrathoracic airway obstruction. Its sudden onset is a terrifying experience for the child and the parents. Inspiratory stridor is the leading symptom for all laryngo-tracheal stenosis. It can occur in both phases of respiration when the obstruction is severe. Most cases of acute stridor are due to laryngotracheobronchitis (croup) caused mainly by parainfluenza viruses type B. Other less common causes include respiratory syncytial virus (RSV), adenoviruses, influenza A and B viruses and measles virus. The infection is usually benign and produces inflammation affecting the larynx, trachea, bronchi and sometimes pulmonary parenchyma. The onset is usually characterised by an URTI, followed by barking cough, hoarseness and a varying degree of respiratory distress. Persistent stridor commencing in the first few weeks of life is mostly caused by laryngomalacia as a result of collapse of the supraglottic structure during inspiration. A child with laryngomalacia has a normal cry (no hoarse voice) and a normal cough.

Possible Diagnoses

Infants	Children
Common	
Laryngomalacia	Laryngotracheobronchitis (croup)
Post-ventilation	Laryngomalacia
Haemangioma	Angioneurotic oedema
Croup	Spasmodic croup
	Bacterial tracheitis
Rare	
Vascular ring	Tonsillar lymphoma
Hypoglycaemia (rickets)	Hypoglycaemia (rickets)
Laryngeal web	Measles croup
Glottic stenosis	Foreign body
Diphtheritic croup	Epiglottitis
Chiari malformation	

Differential Diagnosis at a Glance

	Croup	Spasmodic Croup	Bacterial Tracheitis	Laryngomalacia	Angioedema
Short history	Yes	Yes	Yes	No	Yes
Fever	Possible	No	Yes	No	No
With URTI	Yes	No	Possible	No	No
Onset at night	Yes	Yes	No	No	No
Hoarseness	Yes	Yes	No	No	Possible

Recommended Investigations

Most acute cases of croup do not require any investigation. There is overlap with the investigation in children with hoarseness or stridor (see previous section on hoarseness [dysphonia]).

Top Tips

- History and respiratory sounds do not define the location and the nature of the stenosis. Endoscopy is required to detect the exact location, degree of stenosis, and its relation to other tissues.
- The most important aspect of acute stridor is to differentiate between a life-threatening illness such as epiglottitis or foreign body and a relatively harmless croup caused by a viral infection.
- Nocturnal onset of acute stridor with barking cough and hoarse voice is almost certainly croup, whether viral or spasmodic.
- Laryngomalacia is the most common cause of persistent stridor during infancy. It is caused by a soft tissue laxity above the vocal cords, which collapses during inspiration. Parents can be reassured that recovery will occur when the child is aged 12–18 months, often even earlier.
- Once the diagnosis of laryngomalacia is made, direct examination of the larynx is not indicated.
- Angioedema is either allergic (often with urticaria), idiopathic, or hereditary, which is present with recurrent episodes of swelling caused by mutation of the gene encoding C1 esterase inhibitors. It is non-pitting, non-dependent and transient, which is either histamine-mediated or bradykinin-mediated, which is not mediated by IgE and not associated with urticaria; adrenaline is ineffective.

Red Flags

- A neonate with respiratory distress and severe stridor may have a laryngeal web between the vocal cords. Immediate laryngoscopy is required to prevent asphyxia. Laser treatment is successful.
- A toxic-looking child with high fever and swallowing difficulty has epiglottitis. Admit to intensive care unit (ICU), and consult an ENT surgeon and an anaesthetist. Do not examine the throat as this could cause laryngeal spasm and respiratory obstruction.
- Some children with croup (1%–2%) may present with increasing respiratory distress and worsening tachycardia. They will need intensive care and intubation.
- It is unusual for the common croup to have hypoxia (pulse oximeter below 92%). If present, this would be an ominous sign requiring urgent attention.
- Angioedema is often life-threatening, depending on underlying cause and location. Prompt administration of adrenaline is life-saving, even if it turned out to be bradykinin-mediated.
- Laryngomalacia should be investigated if associated with respiratory distress, dyspnoea, cyanosis, failure to thrive or obstructive sleep disorders.
- In the absence of a viral respiratory tract infection, an acute stridor in an infant or toddler may suggest foreign-body aspiration. This is more likely if the history suggests sudden choking and coughing.

FURTHER READING

Sittel C. Pathologies of the larynx and trachea in children. *GMS Curr Top Otorhinolaryngol Head Neck Surg* 2014;13:Doc09.

SWALLOWING DIFFICULTY (DYSPHAGIA)

Clinical Overview

Swallowing is a complex mechanism involving some 50 muscle pairs (agonists and antagonists) to bring swallowed material to the stomach. Swallowing is observed as early as 20 weeks of gestation with amniotic fluid swallowing. Sucking and swallowing and their coordination are established at 33–34 weeks of gestation. Dysphagia is defined as a difficulty in swallowing due to impaired transfer of fluids or food from the oral cavity to the oesophagus (pre-oesophageal) and from the oesophagus to the stomach (oesophageal dysphagia). Causes of pre-oesophageal dysphagia are mainly neuromuscular, such as bulbar palsy and myasthenia gravis. Dysphagia involves liquids and solids, liquids being more difficult to swallow than solids. Causes of oesophageal dysphagia are in the lumen (stricture, web, tumour, foreign body or ring), in the wall (oesophagitis), or extramural (mediastinal mass). In infants, dysphagia may manifest as low interest in food, body stiffness or vomiting during feeding, unusually lengthy feeding or coughing or gagging during feeding.

Possible Diagnoses

Infants	Children
Common	
Extreme prematurity	Oropharyngeal (e.g. tonsillitis, tonsillar abscess, epiglottitis)
Asphyxia	Neuromuscular (e.g. bulbar palsy in spasticity)
Respiratory distress syndrome	Globus hystericus
Cleft lip and palate	Oesophagitis
Neuromuscular	Collagen vascular diseases (e.g. dermatomyositis)
Rare	
Tracheo-oesophageal fistula	Mediastinal mass
Vascular ring	Neuromuscular (e.g. myasthenia gravis)
Oesophageal stricture	Oesophagitis (GO reflux, corrosive ingestion)
Nasal obstruction (choanal stenosis/atresia)	Oesophageal tumour, web
Prader-Willi syndrome	Oesophageal stricture
	Oesophageal foreign body
	Potocki-Lupski syndrome (chromosomal duplication)
	Ectopic thyroid
	Eosinophilic oesophagitis
	Achalasia
	Vascular ring
	Lower oesophageal ring (Schatzki's ring)
	Plummer-Vinson syndrome (sideropenic dysphagia)
	Oesophageal diverticulum (pharyngeal or oesophageal)
	Drugs (potassium chloride, quinidine)

Differential Diagnosis at a Glance

	Oropharyngeal	Spasticity	Globus Hystericus	Oesophagitis	Collagen Disease
Acute onset	Yes	No	Possible	Possible	No
Fever	Yes	No	No	No	Possible
More solids	Yes	No	Yes	Yes	Yes
Neuro signs	No	Yes	No	No	Possible
Symptom mild	Yes	No	Yes	Possible	Possible

Recommended Investigations

** Serum muscle enzymes (creatine phosphokinase): elevated in some neuromuscular diseases, e.g. dermatomyositis
** Chest X-ray for possible vascular ring or aspiration pneumonia
*** Barium meal for any oesophageal cause of dysphagia, including external compression
*** Oesophagoscopy to identify structural abnormalities or to obtain biopsy
*** pH study to detect GO reflux
** Video-fluoroscopy may detect oesophageal web and motor disorders such as achalasia

Top Tips

- The incidence of feeding/swallowing disorders is increasing due to increased survival of premature babies (up to 80% experience oral feeding difficulty) and improved life expectancy of children with disability.
- A young patient who complains of having a lump in the throat or neck that is unrelated to swallowing is almost certainly experiencing globus hystericus. This usually occurs in association with anxiety, stress or grief.
- Untreated severe iron-deficiency anaemia can cause a thin mucosal membrane that grows across the lumen of the oesophagus.
- Achalasia is a neurogenic oesophageal disorder of unknown aetiology which is characterised by the absence of peristalsis during swallowing. This can be demonstrated by a barium meal.
- Unless the cause of the swallowing difficulty is easily established and acute (e.g. tonsillitis), management is the responsibility of an expert team including a speech-language therapist.

Red Flags

- It is important to treat GO reflux before oesophagitis and stricture develop.
- Infants with swallowing difficulty who are fed by mouth are at a high risk of aspiration which leads to recurrent aspiration pneumonia.
- Children with neuromuscular disorders (e.g. cerebral palsy) are at risk of aspiration-induced lung injury, failure to thrive and social isolation. An early referral to a neurologist and a surgeon for consideration of gastrostomy is indicated.
- Be aware that in children presenting an unexplained respiratory problem, such as persistent cough or aspiration pneumonia, oropharyngeal dysphagia should be considered.

FURTHER READING

Lau C. Development of suck and swallow mechanisms in infants. *Ann Nutr Metab* 2015;66(Suppl 5):7–14.

6 NOSE

NASAL DISCHARGE/BLOCKED NOSE

Clinical Overview

Nasal discharge and blockage are extremely common in children. By far the most common causes are viral infectious rhinitis, allergic rhinitis (more common in older children and adults; Figure 6.1) and adenoid hypertrophy. Breathing difficulty in neonates and young infants may be caused by nasal obstruction as a result of partial or complete choanal atresia. Although the vast majority of causes are benign and self-limiting, serious conditions include nasopharyngeal tumours, encephalocele and foreign body. In these conditions, discharge is usually purulent and foul smelling, with or without blood. Obstruction in the nasal passage normally causes mouth breathing. Exclusively oral breathing is rare or non-existent. It is rather a mixed nasal and mouth breathing. Prolonged mouth breathing may lead to disorder of speech, dental malocclusion and facial deformity (adenoid facies). Nasal discharge/blockage impacts negatively on a child's quality of life by interfering with sleep, daytime activities and school performance. Nasal discharge/blockage may also exert effects on the sinuses, throat and voice that manifest as impaired hearing, worsening asthma and problematic snoring.

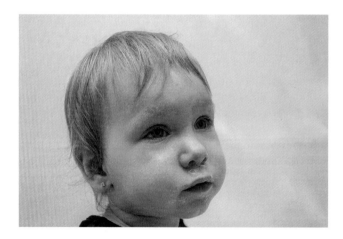

FIGURE 6.1 Nasal discharge and red eyes in allergic rhinitis.

Possible Diagnoses

Infants	Children
Common	
Baby snuffles	Viral infectious rhinitis
Viral infectious rhinitis	Allergic rhinitis (AR)
Adenoid hypertrophy	Adenoid hypertrophy
Congenital narrowing of nasal passages	Vasomotor rhinitis (VR)
Choanal atresia/stenosis	Nasal polyposis

(Continued)

(Continued)

Infants	Children
Rare	
Allergic rhinitis	Foreign body (occurring commonly in toddlers)
Nasal septum deviation (birth trauma)	Nasopharyngeal tumour (e.g. angio-fibroma)
Congenital syphilis	Deviated nasal septum
Hypothyroidism	Unilateral choanal atresia or stenosis
Encephalocele	Hypothyroidism
Immotile cilia syndrome	Drugs causing rhinitis, cocaine abuse
Coloboma, heart defect, atresia rate of the choanae, retarded growth, genital hypoplasia and ear anomaly (CHARGE) syndrome	Immotile cilia syndrome
	Immunodeficiency
	Trauma causing cerebrospinal fluid rhinorrhoea
	Encephalocele

Differential Diagnosis at a Glance

	Upper Respiratory Tract Infection	AR	Adenoid Hypertrophy	VR	Nasal Polyps
Infants affected	Yes	Possible	Yes	No	No
Prolonged symptoms	No	Yes	Yes	No	Yes
Itching/sneezing	Possible	Yes	No	Possible	No
Diagnosis by nasal endoscopy	No	Possible	No	No	Yes
Positive allergy tests	No	Yes	No	No	Possible

Recommended Investigations

*   Full blood count (FBC): the presence of eosinophilia may suggest allergic rhinitis
*** Total IgE in blood, skin prick testing, or blood antibodies for possible allergens
*   Sinus X-ray may identify sinus opacity suggestive of sinusitis or a mass
*** Nasal endoscopy for polyps or tumours
*** Computed tomography (CT) or magnetic resonance imaging is more sensitive than plain X-ray to diagnose sinusitis or a tumour

Top Tips

- Blocked nose in babies ('snuffles') is common due to presence of mucus in a narrowed nasal passage. It is loud during feeding and sleep and disappears when the baby reaches 4–5 months; reassurance is the best medicine.
- Neonates are obligatory nasal breathers; therefore, those with bilateral choanal atresia present with severe respiratory distress and cyanosis that improves when the child cries. Unilateral choanal atresia or stenosis may be asymptomatic for many months and presents later as persistent unilateral nasal discharge or unilateral severe nasal obstruction.
- Atresia or stenosis is diagnosed by inability to pass a nasal catheter 3–4 cm into the nasopharynx.
- Symptoms of VR resemble those of AR but an allergic cause and eosinophils in nasal secretions are absent; itching and sneezing are minimal. Acute nasal obstruction with profuse watery discharge is suggestive of VR.

- It is easy to diagnose polyps. In contrast to the highly vascularised pink turbinate tissue, polyps are a grey, shiny, grape-looking mass present between the nasal turbinates and the septum.

Red Flags

- Choanal atresia is associated with other congenital anomalies in about 50% (e.g. CHARGE syndrome).
- An important cause of 'baby snuffles' is congenital syphilis. Anaemia and splenomegaly are other findings.
- While a foul-smelling or blood-tinged unilateral discharge in a toddler suggests foreign-body aspiration, a persistent bloody discharge always suggests a tumour, including malignancy.
- Although intranasal steroids are the most effective medication available for the treatment of AR, their prolonged use may cause growth suppression and atrophic changes in the nasal mucosa.
- The presence of nasal polyps should lead clinicians to exclude cystic fibrosis (CF), even in the absence of pulmonary or intestinal symptoms. Some 20%–25% of patients with CF have polyps.
- Polyps are more commonly bilateral; if unilateral, benign and malignant tumours should be distinguished by nasal endoscopy, CT scan and/or biopsy.
- Be wary of 'obstructive sleep apnoea' with chronic airway obstruction, including nasal obstruction, which can lead to chronic hypoxia, growth failure, pulmonary hypertension, right-sided heart failure and even death. Predisposing factors include adenotonsillar hypertrophy and trisomy 21.
- Some asthmatic children react with severe dyspnoea and nasal symptoms within 2 hours of aspirin ingestion. An 'aspirin triad' consists of asthma, polyps and aspirin sensitivity.
- Overuse of over-the-counter medications (e.g. nasal spray or decongestants) may lead to rhinitis medicamentosa. Taking a history should include what nasal medications have been used.

FURTHER READING

Basheer B, Hegde KS, Bahat SS et al. Influence of mouth breathing on the dentofacial growth in children: A cephalometric study. *J Int Oral Health* 2014;6(6):50–55.
Meltzer EO, Caballero F, Krouse JH et al. Treatment of congestion in upper respiratory diseases. *Int J Gen Medicine* 2010;3:69–91.

NOSEBLEED (EPISTAXIS)

Clinical Overview

Epistaxis in children is a common condition, which is usually benign and self-limiting but often causes significant parental anxiety. About 30% of children aged under 5 years and over 50% of those aged 6–10 years experience at least one episode of epistaxis. Incidence is rare before 2 years of age and uncommon after puberty. The nasal mucosa of the nasal septum has a rich vascular supply arising from convergence of both internal and external carotid arteries (Kiesselbach's plexus). Epistaxis is classified, on the basis of bleeding site, into anterior and posterior. The majority of bleeds (over 90%) originate from the anterior caudal septum. This location, with its thin mucosa, is predisposed to trauma such as local irritation. Epistaxis may, however, be a sign of serious systemic disease such as coagulopathy or vascular disorder such as hereditary haemorrhagic telangiectasia (HHT). When dealing with severe epistaxis, assessment of the vital signs, airway and circulation stability are more important than the bleeding itself.

Possible Diagnoses

Infants	Children
Common	
Coagulopathy (e.g. vitamin K deficiency)	Digital trauma (e.g. nose picking)
Iatrogenic (e.g. nasogastric tube)	Inflammation (hay fever, infectious rhinitis)
	Coagulopathy
	Foreign body
	Drugs (local decongestant, nasal steroids, cocaine)
	Low ambient humidity
Rare	
HIV	Tumours (e.g. polyps, angio-fibroma)
Congenital vascular abnormalities	Chronic cocaine abuse
Choanal stenosis	Hypertension
	Child abuse (physical abuse <2 years of age)
	Ehlers-Danlos syndrome
	HHT
	Ataxia-telangiectasia
	Migraine

Differential Diagnosis at a Glance

	Trauma	Inflammatory	Coagulopathy	Foreign Body	Drugs
History is diagnostic	Possible	Yes	Yes	Possible	Yes
The only symptom	Yes	Possible	No	Possible	No
Severe epistaxis	Possible	No	Yes	Possible	No
Likely recurrence	Yes	Possible	Yes	No	Possible
Abnormal blood tests	No	No	Yes	No	Possible

Recommended Investigations

*** FBC: to check for haemoglobin in case of massive bleeding; platelet count for thrombocytopenia

*** Coagulation screens with prothrombin time (for vitamin K deficiency), partial thromboplastin time (to screen for haemophilia)

*** Further clotting studies if coagulation screens are abnormal

*** Imaging with CT scan or magnetic resonance imaging for severe and frequent epistaxis

Top Tips

- Epistaxis is usually self-limiting and requires no investigation. Frequent and severe epistaxis should be investigated for an underlying disorder such as coagulopathy or tumour.
- Distinguishing local from systemic causes of epistaxis is essential for applying appropriate therapy. The child should undergo thorough physical examination to exclude systemic disease such as coagulopathy, leukaemia or von Willebrand disease. The parents will appreciate their child's blood pressure being checked as they may consider hypertension to be the cause.
- HHT is autosomal dominant with a prevalence of 1:5,000 people. Telangiectasia can occur on oral or on nasal mucosa, face and fingers.
- In managing epistaxis, the nostrils should be compressed and the child kept in an upright position with the head tilted forward to avoid blood trickling posteriorly in the pharynx. If bleeding stops, the child is sent home after 30 minutes of observation. If not, electro-coagulation or silver nitrate cautery is applied.

Red Flags

- Any epistaxis occurring under the age of 2 years, particularly if severe, requires investigation to exclude systemic diseases, e.g. blood dyscrasia. Urgent referral to an ear, nose and throat specialist is indicated.
- In adolescents with recurrent epistaxis and nasal ulcers, consider the possibility of cocaine use.
- Although laypeople often associate epistaxis with hypertension, this is rarely the case. Be aware, however, that anxiety from having epistaxis may cause mild hypertension.
- Be aware that epistaxis at night may cause swallowing of blood, leading to haematemesis and/or melaena occurring the next morning.
- Epistaxis originating from the posterior bleeding site is uncommon in children and is usually profuse; inflammation or neoplasm should be excluded.
- Be aware that massive epistaxis is often the first and only symptom of HHT before the appearance of the characteristic skin and mucosal membrane lesions (occurring in 80%). Around 20% of patients have pulmonary arteriovenous malformations (AVMs) that may present as stroke due to embolic abscess. Disease complications may result in premature death. Screening for organ involvement is essential (e.g. pulmonary, liver and gastrointestinal AVM).
- Juvenile nasal angiofibroma is a benign tumour of the nasopharynx that usually presents with nasal obstruction and epistaxis. The tumour may be mistaken as a nasal polyp.
- While a foul-smelling or blood-tinged unilateral discharge suggests a foreign body, particularly in toddlers, a persistent bloody discharge always suggests tumour, including malignancy.

FURTHER READING

Beck R, Sorge M, Schneider A et al. General approach to epistaxis treatment in primary and secondary care. *Dtsch Arztebl Int* 2018;115(1–2):12–22.

De Gussem EM, Edwards CP, Hosman AE et al. Life expectancy of patients with hereditary haemorrhagic telangiectasia. *Orphanet J Rare Dis* 2016;11:46.

7 ORAL

BAD BREATH (HALITOSIS)

Clinical Overview

Halitosis (malodour) is the third most frequent reason for attending dental care centres, after tooth decay and gum disease. It is defined as an exhaled air containing more than 75 parts per billion of odour-producing volatile sulphur compounds (VSCs), which are generated by anaerobic bacteria located principally on the back of the tongue. Halitosis is a symptom caused by various conditions including poor oral hygiene, dry mouth, dental diseases (particularly periodontal disease) and gastrointestinal and pulmonary problems. The oral cavity (particularly on the dorsum of the tongue and in areas between teeth) is the most common source of halitosis and is responsible in about 85% of cases. Conditions that predispose to halitosis include decrease in the flow of saliva, a high amount of protein in the diet, a reduced amount of carbohydrates, dental and gum diseases and prolonged intake of antibiotics.

Possible Diagnoses

Infants	Children
Common	
Mouth inflammation	Poor oral hygiene
Dehydration (e.g. fever)	Dehydration (e.g. fever and mouth breathing)
Certain foods (e.g. spices)	Pharyngitis/tonsillitis
Medications	Pseudo-halitosis
Poor dental hygiene	Dental diseases
Oral candidiasis	
Rare	
Gastro-intestinal diseases	Gum diseases
	Medications
	Gastro-oesophageal reflux
	Bronchiectasis
	Eating certain foods (e.g. garlic, spices)
	Nasal foreign body
	Respiratory, liver, renal diseases

Differential Diagnosis at a Glance

	Poor Oral Hygiene	Dehydration	Pharyngitis/Tonsillitis	Pseudo-Halitosis	Dental Diseases
Dry mouth/mucosa	Possible	Yes	Possible	No	Possible
Fever	No	Possible	Yes	No	Possible
Acute onset	No	Possible	Yes	No	Possible
Normal smell	Possible	Possible	Possible	Yes	Possible
Red inflamed mouth	No	Possible	Yes	No	Possible

Recommended Investigations

* Halimeter for measuring the level of VSCs
* OralChroma to detect dimethyl sulphide

Top Tips

• A child presenting with halitosis should be examined by smelling his or her breath from a distance of 10–15 cm. The odour is scored on a five-point scale. The tongue's odour is measured by scraping the back of the tongue with a plastic spoon and evaluating the smell on the spoon.

• Pseudo-halitosis is common and occurs when halitosis does not actually exist but parents (and sometimes children themselves) perceive it as such. Reassurance is all that is needed.

• While the Halimeter can detect VSCs for oral halitosis, the OralChroma can detect dimethyl sulphide (produced during fermentation of beer) for extra-oral halitosis.

• Some medications (e.g. antihistamines, anti-cholinergics) may cause dry mouth (xerostomia) with its complications such as taste alteration, dental caries and halitosis. Other medications (e.g. chloral hydrate, paraldehyde, cytotoxic drugs) are directly the cause of halitosis.

• The Halimeter is a useful device to confirm halitosis; the measurement involves a flexible straw being inserted in the mouth or nostril while the patient holds his or her breath. The measurement is in parts per billion and any measurement more than 75 per billion is diagnostic.

• Be aware that the coating on the tongue is often the cause of halitosis. Gentle daily cleaning of the dorsum of the tongue is recommended. Oral hygiene is essential with toothbrushing and mouthwash (e.g. with chlorhexidine). If xerostomia exists, plenty of sugar-free fluids may stimulate the salivary flow.

Red Flags

• Remember that fever is the most common cause of dry mouth because of increased insensible perspiration. Extra cups of fluids are beneficial for both the fever and the halitosis.

• Be aware that halitosis may be a clue to some serious underlying cause such as bronchiectasis or nasal foreign body.

• Unexplained oral and dental trauma may be caused by physical and/or sexual child abuse. Manifestations include oral bruising, abrasions and laceration of the tongue, lips and frenum. Other features that may be caused by sexual abuse include oral erythema, vesicles and ulcer.

• If a Halimeter is used to diagnose halitosis, make sure the device is specific for VSCs, not for dimethyl sulphide, which also produces odour detectable by another device (OralChroma).

FURTHER READING

Bakhtiari S, Senatpour M, Mortazavi H et al. Oro-facial manifestations of adverse reactions: A review study. *Clujul Med* 2018;91(1):27–36.
Costacurta M, Benavoli D, Arcudi G et al. Oral and dental signs of child abuse and neglect. *Oral Implantol (Rome)* 2015;8(2–3):68–73.

DENTAL CARIES

Clinical Overview

Dental caries is the most common chronic infectious disease of childhood caused by the interaction of bacteria (mainly *Streptococcus mutans*) and sugary foods on tooth enamel (Figure 7.1). These bacteria break down sugars, causing an acidic environment in the oral cavity, resulting in demineralisation of the tooth enamel and dental caries. The length of time of exposure of the teeth to sugars is the crucial factor in the aetiology of dental caries. The World Health Organisation recommends the intake of sugar should provide less than 10% of energy intake, and even less than 5% of energy, to protect dental health throughout life. Acids produced by bacteria after sugar intake persist for 20–40 minutes. Dental caries cause pain, anxiety, time lost at school, hospitalisation and negative impact on life, and are costly to the healthcare system. Risk factors for dental caries include genetic and racial factors, unavailability of water fluoride, poor oral hygiene including toothbrushing, poverty, low level of education and malocclusion of the teeth.

Possible Diagnoses

Infants	Children
Common	
Early childhood caries (ECC)	ECC
Incipient caries	Incipient caries
	Arrested caries
	Recurrent caries
	Rampant caries

Differential Diagnosis at a Glance

	ECC	Incipient Caries	Arrested Caries	Recurrent Caries	Rampant Caries
Infants/toddlers	Yes	Yes	Possible	Possible	No
Related to bottle feeding	Yes	Possible	Possible	Possible	No
Previous history of caries	No	No	Possible	Yes	Possible
Related to oral hygiene	No	No	Possible	Possible	Yes
Drug related	No	No	Possible	Possible	Yes

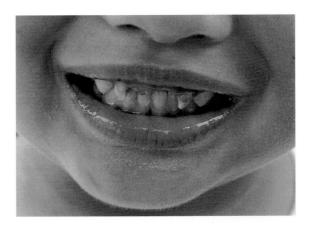

FIGURE 7.1 Caries and tooth decay.

Recommended Investigations

* Dental X-ray

Top Tips

- ECC is defined as the presence of one or more decayed, missing or filled tooth surface in any primary tooth in children younger than 6 years of age. Arrested caries is a caries that was previously demineralised but later re-mineralised before the cavity is formed. Rampant caries is a severe form of caries affecting multiple surfaces and many teeth. It is associated with dry mouth, poor oral hygiene and drugs such as amphetamine.
- ECC is identified as a white band of demineralised enamel that quickly advances to obvious decay along the gingival margin.
- There is a positive correlation between dental caries and body mass index (BMI). The lifestyle of obese children, including sugary snack and soda taking, predisposes to dental caries later on in life. Malnutrition causes decreased flow of the salivary glands that predisposes to dental caries.
- Sugars of grains, fruits, vegetables and milk do not contribute to the development of dental caries because of these items' intrinsic structures. They also stimulate the salivary flow that eliminates the sugars. The main cause of dental caries is the free sugars that include monosaccharides (glucose, galactose, fructose) and disaccharides added to the food by the manufacturer or consumed as syrup, honey and fruit juices.
- The best available evidence for the role of sugar in causing dental caries comes from those countries which have low dental caries when the free sugars are kept low (40–55 g/person/day).

Red Flags

- Even mild dental caries in children is of concern because it is a lifelong progressive disease.
- Early caries can be a particularly virulent form of caries, beginning soon after dental eruption, progressing rapidly and having a lasting impact on both primary and permanent dentition.
- A decline in dental caries rates was found until the mid-1980s; recently a reverse has been reported.

FURTHER READING

Moynihan P. Sugars and dental caries: Evidence for setting a recommended threshold for intake. *Adv Nutr* 2016;7(1):149–156.
Hooley M, Skouteris M, Cecile B et al. Body mass index and dental caries in children and adolescents: A systematic review of literature published 2004 to 2011. *Syst Rev* 2012;1:57.

MOUTH BLEEDING

Clinical Overview

Mouth bleeding is common in the paediatric population. It is usually mild, not life-threatening and the cause is usually found locally. However, it is distressing for the parents to witness. The most common cause is trauma such as cutting the lip or mouth as a result of a fall or running into a solid object. Another common cause is epistaxis dripping down the throat. Periodontal diseases (affecting the gingiva, alveolar bone, cementum and periodontal ligament) are other important causes of bleeding. Extra-oral causes of mouth bleeding are uncommon and include serious underlying systemic disorders such as thrombocytopenia, leukaemia, aplastic anaemia and von Willebrand disease. These are particularly important if there is no obvious local cause for the bleeding.

Possible Diagnoses

Infants	Children
Common	
Trauma (including birth trauma)	Trauma
Candidiasis	Gingivitis
Liver cholestasis	Immune thrombocytopenia (ITP)
Coagulopathy (e.g. haemophilia)	Nosebleed
Vitamin K deficiency (breastfed infants)	Periodontitis
Rare	
Neonatal thrombocytopenia	Drugs (e.g. methotrexate, aspirin)
	Von Willebrand disease
	Scurvy
	Child abuse
	Hepatic failure
	Haemophilia
	Hereditary haemorrhagic telangiectasia

Differential Diagnosis at a Glance

	Trauma	Gingivitis	Thrombocytopenia	Nosebleed	Periodontitis
Purpura on skin	Possible	No	Possible	No	No
Large bleed	Possible	No	Possible	Possible	No
Diagnosis by history	Possible	Possible	Possible	Possible	No
Oral inflammatory changes	Possible	Yes	No	No	Yes
Associated pain	Yes	Possible	No	No	Possible

Recommended Investigations

For systemic extra-oral causes of bleeding:

- *** Full blood count (FBC): to exclude thrombocytopenia, aplastic anaemia
- *** First-stage tests: prothrombin time, partial thromboplastin time, bleeding and clotting time; second-stage tests: von Willebrand factor, fibrinogen and thrombin
- *** Liver function test for suspected liver disease

Top Tips

- Bleeding from vitamin K deficiency usually occurs within the first 1–7 days of life and rarely as late as 12 weeks. Entirely breastfed infants have a 20 times greater risk of such deficiency than those receiving formula.
- Bleeding from the gum or gingivitis is usually due to poor oral hygiene. Prevention of bleeding rests on promoting proper oral hygiene, e.g. regular teeth brushing and use of dental floss.
- The absence of a local source of bleeding in the mouth is a very important clue for the presence of extra-oral sources such as thrombocytopenia, von Willebrand disease or leukaemia.
- ITP and von Willebrand disease are among the most common haematological problems affecting children. Affected children often present with oral bleeding.
- Oropharyngeal candidiasis does not bleed unless the white plaque is removed from the underlying tissue, leaving pinpoint haemorrhages.

Red Flags

- Blood from a nosebleed may flow down the throat and be mistakenly considered as a mouth bleed.
- Be aware of melaena caused by continuous swallowing of oral bleeding that has gone unnoticed.
- Be aware that haematemesis may be caused by the swallowing of blood from mouth bleeding.
- Child abuse should always be considered as a possible cause if an infant or young child presents with unexplained mouth injury or the injury is not compatible with the history given. In such a case the skin should be examined for bruises; skeletal survey may be necessary.
- Gingivitis with mouth bleeding may be the presenting symptom of acute non-lymphoblastic leukaemia, thrombocytopenia or neutropenia. Early diagnosis is crucial.

FURTHER READING

McIntosh N. Incidence of oronasal haemorrhage in infancy presenting to general practice in the UK. *Br J Gen Pract* 2008;58(557):877–879.

MOUTH ULCERS

Clinical Overview

Mouth ulceration is common in children. It may be caused by trauma (physical or chemical), viral infections, aphthous ulcers, dermatological or haematopoietic disorders, gastrointestinal disease, nutritional deficiency or as a side effect of drugs. Most acute mouth ulcers in young children (Figure 7.2) are caused by viral infection, such as acute herpetic gingivostomatitis (AHG), or trauma. Aphthous ulcers are more common in older children and adults (affecting about 20% of the population), with a tendency to recur in contrast to AHG. The appearance of mouth ulcers may be quite challenging as they may be caused by serious systemic diseases such as inflammatory bowel diseases, lymphoproliferative diseases, neutropenia, syphilis and juvenile-onset systemic lupus erythematosus (SLE).

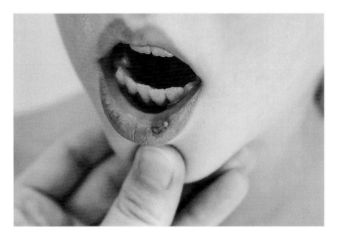

FIGURE 7.2   Gingivostomatitis.

Possible Diagnoses

Infants	Children
Common	
AHG	AHG
Medications	Hand-foot-mouth disease
Trauma (including child abuse)	Herpangina
Exanthem (e.g. varicella, measles)	Trauma (including child abuse, chemical burns)
Neutropenia	Aphthous ulcers
Rare	
Periodic fever syndrome (e.g. periodic fever, aphthous stomatitis, pharyngitis and cervical adenitis [PFAPA])	Other viral infections (e.g. EBV)
Hand-foot-mouth disease	Inflammatory bowel disease (e.g. Crohn's disease)
Neonatal lupus	Neutropenia (cyclic, aplastic anaemia)
Neonatal syphilis	Lichen planus
Nutrient deficiencies	Fungal infection
	Erythema multiforme
	Medications (e.g. chemotherapy)

(*Continued*)

(Continued)

Infants	Children
	Facial herpes zoster
	Histoplasmosis
	HIV infection
	Tuberculosis
	Acute necrotising ulcerative gingivitis (ANUG)
	Periodic fever syndrome (e.g. PFAPA)
	Behçet's disease
	Oral sarcoidosis
	SLE
	Stevens-Johnson syndrome
	Nutrient deficiencies (e.g. vitamin B_{12})
	Coeliac disease
	Lymphoproliferative diseases, mouth cancer
	Reiter's syndrome (uveitis, conjunctivitis, arthritis)

Differential Diagnosis at a Glance

	AHG	Hand-Foot-Mouth	Herpangina	Trauma	Aphthous Ulcers
Fever	Yes	Possible	Yes	No	No
Affect the gingiva	Yes	Possible	No	Possible	Possible
Size <10 mm	Yes	Yes	Yes	Possible	Possible
History of recurrence	No	No	No	Possible	Yes
Extra-oral sites	No	Yes	No	Possible	No

Recommended Investigations

*** FBC: cyclic neutropenia, anaemia in Crohn's disease; leukopenia, anaemia and thrombocytopenia in SLE

*** C-reactive protein: elevated in bacterial infectious disease

*** Serological tests for HIV infection

** Dark field microscopy from debris obtained from ANUG lesions will demonstrate spirochetes

** Scraping for culture in suspected fungal infection; if positive, tests for immunity

Top Tips

- Benign aphthae tend to be small in size (<1 cm) and self-limiting in about 90% of cases, while large aphthae are often associated with more serious disorders such as HIV infection.
- The presence of pain can be a helpful marker diagnostically: AHG, traumatic and aphthous ulcers are painful; ulcers caused by SLE and lymphoproliferative diseases are painless.
- Differentiating herpangina from AHG is usually easy: herpangina has more posterior lesions (tonsils, tonsillar pillars, uvula, pharyngeal wall and soft palate), while in AHG the lesions affect the cheeks, gingiva and tongue.
- ANUG is rare in healthy children but may occur in association with malnutrition and poor oral hygiene. It is very painful, distinguishing it from the common usually painless chronic gingivitis. There is also bleeding and ulceration. It may mimic AHG. It can be caused by spirochetes, and dark field microscopy will detect them.
- Episodes of PFAPA are characterised by attacks of unprovoked systemic inflammation with periodic fever. Each episode is followed by a symptom-free interval ranging in duration from weeks to months. Steroids are effective therapy.

Red Flags

- A child with atopic dermatitis who becomes infected with herpes virus resulting in eczema herpeticum needs care. This is the most serious manifestation of herpes virus and may be lethal.
- Mouth ulcers are common in Crohn's disease, but rare in ulcerative colitis. Beware that the mouth lesions may precede the intestinal manifestations (prevalence estimated 20%–50%).
- Multiple mouth ulcers may be the first sign of neutropenia or aplastic anaemia.
- Major aphthae, which are difficult to heal, need dental consultation to exclude more serious diseases such as HIV. Other manifestations of HIV include oral candidiasis and periodontitis.
- Initial symptoms and signs of leukaemia may appear in the mouth due to leukaemic cell infiltration or associated decrease of bone marrow elements such as low white blood cell or platelet counts.
- Beware of oral manifestations of child abuse. These may include broken teeth, lip injury or tears to the lingual frenum. Abuse should be considered if the injury is not compatible with the history.
- Oral gels, which are used to treat oral ulcers, may contain salicylate salts. They should not be given to children under 12 years of age as they may cause Reye's syndrome.

FURTHER READING

Mortazavi H, Safi Y, Baharrand M et al. Diagnostic features of common oral ulcerative lesions: An update decision tree. *Int J Dent* 3 October 2016. doi: 10.1155/2016/7278925

8 EAR

DEAFNESS/IMPAIRED HEARING

Clinical Overview

Hearing impairment is either sensorineural or conductive. Conductive hearing impairment is common: At least half of preschool children have one or more episodes of otitis media with effusion (OME), which is often a cause of varying degrees of hearing impairment, usually mild (26–40 dB). The incidence of congenital sensorineural is approximately 1:1,000 in neonates, usually severe (50–70 dB) or profound (>70 dB). Cytomegalovirus (CMV) is the leading non-genetic cause of this type of hearing loss. Risk factors include genetic hearing loss, low gestation (<32 weeks), pre-auricular pits or tags, branchial cysts, heterochromia of the iris, prolonged jaundice, ototoxic drugs, hypoxic ischaemic encephalopathy, congenital infections (CMV, rubella, syphilis) and neonatal meningitis.

Possible Diagnoses

Infants	Children
Common	
Congenital	OME (glue ears)
Birth asphyxia	Infection (e.g. following meningitis)
Drugs (ototoxic)	Trauma (including acoustic trauma)
Low gestation (<32 weeks)	Drugs (ototoxic drugs)
Bacterial infection (e.g. meningitis)	Genetic
Viral infection (e.g. cytomegalovirus)	CMV
Cleft palate	
Rare	
Microtia	Acoustic neuroma
Tumour	Osteopetrosis
Foreign body	Histiocytosis
	Pendred syndrome
	Osteogenesis imperfecta
	Lyme disease
	Waardenburg syndrome
	Alport syndrome
	Otosclerosis (autosomal dominant)
	HIV infection

Differential Diagnosis at a Glance

	OME	Genetic	Trauma	Drugs	Post-Infection
Severe/profound	No	Yes	Possible	Yes	Possible
Congenital	No	Yes	No	No	No
Likely onset in special care baby unit	No	No	No	Yes	Possible
Abnormal examination finding	Yes	No	Yes	No	No
Detected by screen	No	Yes	No	Possible	Possible

Recommended Investigations

** Tympanogram: if flat, is likely to indicate significant effusion in the middle ear
** Pure-tone audiogram: for more mature and cooperative children

Top Tips

- As parents may not recognise mild or high-frequency hearing impairment and as hearing impairment has a major impact on the child's language and communication, screening testing during the neonatal period is strongly advocated, and usually performed by the third day of life.
- Any child with congenital deafness should be tested for CMV infection as this infection is the leading non-genetic cause of hearing loss.
- The most popular screening is evoked otoacoustic emissions (EOAE), which is inexpensive and the results are easy to interpret. However, it has a high failure rate (about 40%) for days 1 and 2 of life.
- Children who fail the EOAE test or those at risk (e.g. family history, intrauterine infection or craniofacial anomalies) must be evaluated by ABR (auditory brainstem response).
- Although most OME are transient, some children (e.g. those with Down syndrome or cleft palate) are at high risk of developing persistent effusion.
- Although the insertion of grommets for OME is effective in improving language acquisition, this effect lasts as long as the grommets are patent. Long-term benefits are not certain. Antibiotics, antihistamines, decongestants and steroids are usually ineffective.

Red Flags

- Congenital deafness due to congenital infection or genetically determined impairment may escape neonatal screening testing and deteriorate during the first 2 years of life.
- A child with unilateral progressive deafness, vertigo and tinnitus should be suspected as having acoustic neuroma. Children with neurofibromatosis are at higher risk of developing this tumour.
- For any child who presents with psychosocial problems (e.g. hyperactivity and conduct problems) or delayed language and communication, a hearing test is essential.
- When parents suspect that their child's hearing is inadequate or delayed, this must be taken seriously. A rapid referral to an audiological centre should be made.
- Although OME is common, it reduces the conduction sounds entering the ear for up to 40 dB, thus delaying the crucial years of language acquisition.
- An 18-month-old child who has not said a single word with meaning or a 24-month-old child with a single-word vocabulary of less than 10 words should be referred for audiological assessment.
- Exposure to high-intensity sound (80–100 dB in rock music) can cause temporary hearing loss. Sudden and very loud sound >140 dB (gunfire, bombs) may cause permanent hearing loss after one exposure.

FURTHER READING

Hogan SC, Moore DR. Impaired binaural hearing in children produced by a threshold level of middle ear disease. *J Assoc Res Otolaryngol* 2003;4(2):123–129.

DIZZINESS AND VERTIGO

Clinical Overview

Dizziness is difficult to differentiate from vertigo in young children, so the two conditions are joined in this section. Dizziness refers to a sensation of unsteadiness without the perception that the surroundings are rotating. Orthostatic hypotension is a prototype of this category. In true vertigo (such as vestibular neuritis) an older child not only complains of instability, but also has the feeling of spinning or turning. A young child with vertigo is usually noted to appear pale and frightened and/ or suddenly fall onto the ground, losing balance, stumbling or being clumsy. There is no associated hearing loss. The underlying cause is in the equilibratory pathway (vestibule, semicircular canals, eighth nerve, vestibular nuclei in the brainstem and eyes). Vertigo is not a common complaint in children, in contrast to adults. Fortunately, most causes of childhood vertigo are self-limiting.

Possible Diagnoses

Infants	Children
Common	
Physiological (10–18 months of age)	Benign paroxysmal vertigo of childhood (BPVC)
Cerebral degeneration	Acute middle ear disease/eustachian tube dysfunction
Drugs (e.g. sedative, antihistamine)	Vestibular neuritis
Middle ear infection	Labyrinthitis
	Migraine
Rare	
Cerebellar tumour	Orthostatic hypotension (not true vertigo)
	Head injury
	Eustachian tube disease
	Tumours (acoustic neuroma, cerebellar)
	Hypoglycaemia
	Psychogenic
	Fistula between the middle and inner ear
	Chronic otitis media (OM), mastoiditis
	Drugs (e.g. antidepressants, antihistamines)
	Epilepsy (temporal lobe epilepsy)
	Cholesteatoma
	Benign paroxysmal positional vertigo (BPPV)
	Ménière's disease
	Epidemic vertigo (caused by a virus, following upper respiratory tract infection [URTI])

Differential Diagnosis at a Glance

	BPVC	Middle Ear Disease	Vestibular Neuritis	Migraine	Labyrinthitis
True vertigo	Yes	Possible	Yes	Yes	Yes
Paroxysmal	Yes	No	Yes	Yes	Yes
Nystagmus	Yes	No	Yes	Yes	Yes
Fever	No	Yes	No	No	Possible
Hearing loss	No	Possible	No	No	Yes

Recommended Investigations

** Audiogram to assess the ear function
** Tympanometry to evaluate ear function
** Electroencephalogram if there is a suspicion of epilepsy, such as loss of consciousness
** Cranial MRI if trigeminal neuralgia is suspected
** Ice water caloric testing to confirm the abnormal vestibular function
** Cranial MRI to assess for an intracranial lesion

Top Tips

- Testing the vestibular nerve (VN) is done by holding the child in the arms and rotating him or her clockwise and anticlockwise. The normal eye deviation in the direction of rotation and nystagmus in the opposite direction is absent in case of VN dysfunction.
- BPPV and Ménière's disease are the most common causes of vertigo in adults. In children, BPVC, vestibular migraine and vestibular neuritis are the most common causes of vertigo.
- BPVC is characterised by recurrent attacks of vertigo occurring without warning and resolving spontaneously. It is considered as a migraine precursor. Attacks occur mainly in toddlers and are usually triggered by sudden change of the head. After a few seconds there is a sudden onset of pallor, unsteadiness, crying for help, clinging to the mother, or refusing to walk, often with vomiting and horizontal nystagmus. Episodes may last up to 30 seconds and recur in days or weeks.
- Currently, BPPV, benign paroxysmal torticollis, cyclic vomiting and abdominal migraine are identified as periodic syndromes and precursors of migraine.
- Vestibular migraine is a common cause of episodic vertigo combining typical symptoms of migraine with vestibular signs (imbalance, tinnitus, nystagmus) lasting 5 minutes to 72 hours.
- The most common cause of dizziness in young children is middle ear/eustachian tube dysfunction; in older children and adolescents it is orthostatic hypotension, which manifests as feeling unsteady or fainting when getting up from sleep or long sitting.
- Unless the cause of the vertigo is clear (e.g. OM, BPVC), close cooperation between different specialists (e.g. otologist, neurologist, sometimes ophthalmologist and psychiatrist) is essential to establish early diagnosis and management.

Red Flags

- In a child presenting with unremitting vertigo and nystagmus, check for deafness and neurological signs to exclude acoustic neuroma or cerebral degenerative disease.
- Any history of impaired or loss of consciousness in association with vertigo should alert the clinician that the attack could be epileptic (temporal lobe epilepsy).
- Be aware that a young child with BPVC may not complain of dizziness but rather express fear and become pale, unsteady and clumsy.

FURTHER READING

Gasani AP, Dallan I, Navari E et al. Vertigo in children: Proposal for diagnostic algorithm based upon clinical experience. *Acta Otorhinolaryngol Ital* 2015;35(3):180–185.
Tatli B, Gueler S. Non-epileptic events in childhood. *Turk Pediatr Ars* 2017;52(2):59–65.

EARACHE (OTALGIA)

Clinical Overview

This is one of the most common reasons for seeking medical attention. The pain usually arises from inflammation in the middle or external canal of the ear. In infancy, the pain usually manifests as irritability and tenderness when the ear is rubbed or touched. In contrast to adults, referred pain from outside the ears is common in paediatrics, occurring via five main sources: the trigeminal nerve (sensory distribution of the face); the facial nerve (teeth, most commonly the upper molars or temporomandibular joint); the glossopharyngeal nerve (tonsillitis, pharyngitis); the vagus nerve (laryngopharynx or oesophagus); or second to third cervical vertebrae. In these cases patients have a normal otological examination.

Possible Diagnoses

Infants	Children
Common	
Infective OM	Infective OM
Infective otitis externa	Infective otitis externa
Trauma (cauliflower ear)	Referred pain (toothache, tonsillopharyngitis)
Barotitis media (aerotitis)	Trauma (including foreign body)
Infected eczematous dermatitis	Barotitis media (e.g. flying)
Rare	
Furunculosis	Cholesteatoma
Acute cellulitis of the auricle	Mastoiditis
	Trigeminal neuralgia
	Temporomandibular arthritis
	Ramsay Hunt syndrome (herpes zoster oticus)
	Perichondritis/chondritis
	Bullous myringitis
	Exostoses and osteoma
	Impacted cerumen

Differential Diagnosis at a Glance

	Infective OM	Infective External Otitis (EO)	Referred Pain	Trauma	Barotitis
Fever	Yes	Possible	Possible	No	No
Associated URTI	Yes	No	No	No	No
Abnormal eardrum	Yes	No	No	No	No
Being infant	Yes	Possible	Possible	Possible	Possible
Tender on touch	Possible	Yes	No	Possible	No

Recommended Investigations

*   Full blood count: leukocytosis >15,000 may suggest bacterial infection, including occult infection
*** If ear discharge is present, a swab is indicated to identify the organism
*** X-ray and/or CT of the mastoid bone to exclude mastoiditis

Top Tips

- When a child presents with otalgia in one ear, always examine first the ear that does not hurt.
- While perichondritis indicates infection of the surrounding tissue of the auricular cartilage (the outer third of the ear canal), chondritis indicates infection of the cartilage itself. This is usually caused by trauma, such as ear piercing.
- Barotitis occurs through damage to the middle ear due to ambient pressure changes. This may occur during a sudden ambient pressure increase following descent of an airplane or deep sea diving in the presence of dysfunctional eustachian tube by URTI.
- Ramsay Hunt syndrome usually presents with severe ear pain. Vesicles on the pinna and in the external auditory canal in the distribution of the sensory branch of the facial nerve are seen.
- Note that furunculosis, caused by *Staphylococcus aureus* infection, can affect only the cartilaginous outer hair-containing third of the ear.

Red Flags

- The tympanic membrane of a crying baby is often red on inspection; do not misdiagnose OM.
- In neonates, trauma to the pinna may present as haematoma with evolution to cauliflower ear. Immediate needle aspiration of the haematoma is necessary to prevent perichondritis, which can be refractory.
- Infection of the middle ear nowadays is usually caused by a viral infection. Simple pain relievers such as paracetamol or ibuprofen can provide relief. Do not give aspirin!
- Ramsay Hunt syndrome, caused by herpes zoster virus, often causes hearing loss and facial palsy and may be permanent (in 50%). In immunocompromised individuals, infection is serious.
- Remember that some topical otic preparations (neomycin, colistin, polymyxin), used to treat OE, can cause contact dermatitis which manifests as erythema, vesiculation and oedema.
- Parents should be advised to be cautious flying if their child has an URTI or allergy as the relative negative pressure in the middle ear may result in retraction of the tympanic membrane, causing pain and possibly bleeding in the middle ear.

FURTHER READING

Minovi A, Dazert S. Diseases of the middle ear in childhood. *GMC Curr Top Otorhinolaryngol Head Neck Surg* 2014;13:Doc11.

EAR DISCHARGE

Clinical Overview

OM is the most common cause of ear discharge in paediatrics. Its occurrence has become a less seen symptom in recent years mainly because of widespread vaccination, effective antibiotics and better living standards. Children are at high risk for OM and ear discharge if they are in a smoking environment, attend a day care centre, have frequent colds or have allergic rhinitis or adenoid hypertrophy. Risk factors in neonates include nasotracheal intubation for more than 7 days, cleft palate and prematurity. Any ear discharge has to be differentiated from earwax (light, dark or orange brown, normal odour) and water that entered the ear canal during showering or swimming.

Possible Diagnoses

Infants	Children
Common	
Suppurative otitis media	Suppurative OM
Infective otitis externa	Infective otitis external
Haemorrhagic diathesis (disseminated intravascular coagulation)	Seborrhoeic dermatitis
	Otorrhoea from tympanostomy tube
	Trauma
Rare	
Congenital cholesteatoma	Acquired cholesteatoma
	Infected foreign body
	Otorrhoea (cerebrospinal fluid [CSF])
	Herpes zoster
	Mastoiditis
	Tumour (e.g. rhabdomyosarcoma, eosinophilic granuloma)

Differential Diagnosis at a Glance

	OM	OE	Seborrhoeic Dermatitis	Otorrhoea Ear Tube	Trauma
Fever	Yes	Possible	No	No	No
Associated URTI	Yes	No	No	No	No
Purulent	Yes	Yes	No	Yes	No
Normal eardrum	No	Yes	Yes	Yes	Possible
Associated skin lesions	No	No	Yes	No	No

Recommended Investigations

*** Culture of the infected discharge to identify the organisms

** High-resolution computed tomography (HRCT) or MRI if the symptom persists

Top Tips

- Current clinical studies do not recommend immediate antibiotic therapy in most children with uncomplicated OM. Therapy is indicated for children younger than 6 months, moderate to severe otalgia and fever >39.0°C, persistent otorrhoea and high-risk individuals (e.g. Down's syndrome).
- After an acute OM, about 40% of children develop OME that persists for a month; 10% have a persistent OME after 3 months.
- Following tympanostomy tube insertion for OME, at least 50% of children develop otorrhoea through the tube while the tube is properly in place and patent.
- The most serious complication of OM is intracranial suppurative infections including meningitis, subdural empyema and otogenic brain abscess.
- Otitis externa (OE), also called swimmer's ear, tends to recur in children who swim. Instillation of 2% acetic acid immediately after swimming is the most effective prevention. During and after an acute OE, children should not swim and the ears should be protected from water during bathing.

Red Flags

- If otorrhoea persists despite adequate antibiotic cover, cholesteatoma or rhabdomyosarcoma should be suspected. Hearing loss and facial palsy are often present.
- Clear discharge from the ear may be CSF resulting from basilar skull fracture or inner ear malformation. This otogenic CSF leak is potentially life-threatening because of meningitis risk.
- Bloody discharge may follow a direct trauma; a foreign object in the ear canal and, rarely, a tumour should be excluded.
- Foreign-body insertion into the ear is common. Its extraction by a non-otolaryngologist is associated with numerous complications such as eardrum perforation and hearing loss, unless it is easily graspable.

FURTHER READING

Olajuyin O, Olatunja OS. Aural foreign body extraction in children: A double-edged sword. *Pan Afr Med J* 2015;20:186.

9 EYE

Clinical Overview

Acute red eye is common and caused by a variety of conditions including trauma such as a foreign body (FB), diseases of the conjunctiva (conjunctivitis), cornea (keratitis), iris, ciliary body and choroid (uveitis), aqueous humour (glaucoma) and sclera (scleritis and episcleritis). Clinicians should be able to diagnose most common eye diseases, which include allergic conjunctivitis (often seasonal with significant itching, runny nose, swollen lids and positive family history; Figure 9.1), and viral conjunctivitis (with its redness all over the conjunctiva, watery discharge often beginning in one eye, usually caused by adenovirus). Bacterial conjunctivitis is commonly caused by chlamydia in neonates and by staphylococci in older children. It usually produces redness, maximal at the inferior conjunctiva, and purulent discharge or keratitis with redness surrounding the cornea. Any eye redness in neonates or infants requires the exclusion of nasolacrimal duct obstruction and subconjunctival haemorrhage, which may result from injury, inflammation, severe straining, sneezing or coughing. Referral to an ophthalmologist is indicated whenever the diagnosis is unclear.

Possible Diagnoses

Infants	Children
Common	
Lacrimal duct obstruction	Viral conjunctivitis
Chlamydia conjunctivitis	Bacterial conjunctivitis
Episcleral haemorrhage during birth	Allergic conjunctivitis
Chemical conjunctivitis	Keratitis (e.g. herpetic keratitis, contact lens keratitis)
Bacterial conjunctivitis	Trauma (e.g. FB)
Rare	
Gonococcal conjunctivitis	Conjunctivitis associated with systemic diseases
Allergic conjunctivitis	Acute uveitis
Dacryocystitis	Dacryocystitis
	Chemical conjunctivitis
	Epidemic keratoconjunctivitis (EKC)
	Haemorrhagic conjunctivitis
	Glaucoma
	Endophthalmitis (a bacterial infection)
	Vernal conjunctivitis
	Syphilitic interstitial keratitis
	Haemorrhagic conjunctivitis (e.g. caused by picornavirus)
	Biotinidase deficiency (resulting in biotin deficiency)
	Cogan's syndrome (interstitial keratitis with hearing loss)
	Membranous and pseudo-membranous conjunctivitis
	Chalazion and hordeolum

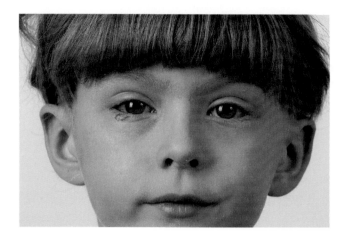

FIGURE 9.1   Conjunctivitis.

Differential Diagnosis at a Glance

	Viral Conjunctivitis	Bacterial Conjunctivitis	Allergic Conjunctivitis	Keratitis	Trauma
Unilateral	Possible	Possible	Yes	Possible	No
Blurred vision	No	No	No	Yes	Possible
Associated pain	No	Possible	No	Yes	Yes
Discharge	Yes	Yes	No	Yes	Possible
Itchy	No	No	Yes	Possible	Possible

Recommended Investigations

If the diagnosis of conjunctivitis in children is clear, laboratory testing, such as culture, is usually not necessary as conjunctivitis is common and harmless. Infection of the cornea by herpes virus produces branch-like (dendritic) lesions, which are demonstrated by fluorescein staining.

- ✱✱ Full blood count (FBC): leukocytosis for bacterial infection
- ✱✱ Anti-nuclear antibodies (ANA) and rheumatoid factor for children with rheumatoid arthritis
- ✱✱✱ Swab for purulent and severe discharge to exclude chlamydia or gonococcal infection
- ✱✱✱ Imaging of the orbit with magnetic resonance imaging (MRI) for any tumour such as rhabdomyosarcoma
- ✱✱✱ Tonometry to measure eye pressure for suspected glaucoma

Top Tips

- Episcleral and retinal haemorrhages in neonates are common after vaginal delivery. Although these seem alarming to parents and clinicians, they are harmless and disappear within 2 weeks.
- Ophthalmia neonatorum refers to inflammation of the conjunctiva within the first month of life. Once principally caused by gonococcal infection, the most common causes are now chlamydia, staphylococci and chemical conjunctivitis caused by the topical antimicrobial

agent silver nitrate. The latter agent reduced the incidence of gonococcal ophthalmia from 10% to 0.3% in 1881.
- At birth, the nasolacrimal duct is often blocked, and the diagnosis is made by the history or by refluxing discharge with a pressure over the lacrimal sac. This resolves spontaneously in more than 95% over a few months, rarely delayed until the age of 1 year and rarely needing surgery.
- Gonococcal conjunctivitis presents in the first few days of life with a rapidly progressive profuse purulent discharge. The cornea is rapidly affected. Urgent treatment with antibiotics is needed.
- Measurement of visual acuity is needed for keratitis, not for conjunctivitis.
- Uveitis presents with pain, lacrimation, photophobia and conjunctival hyperaemia. It occurs mainly in children with a mono-articular or pauci-articular form of rheumatoid arthritis.
- Children with glaucoma usually present with corneal irritation (tearing, photophobia), conjunctival injection and visual impairment. The most important sign is corneal enlargement.
- Systemic diseases associated with conjunctivitis include Kawasaki disease, Stevens-Johnson syndrome and Lyme disease. They are characterised by greater bulbar than palpebral involvement and no eye discharge. In contrast, infectious conjunctivitis has more palpebral involvement.

Red Flags

- Conjunctivitis in neonates may be caused by sexually transmitted diseases acquired during vaginal delivery. Ensure you do not miss chlamydia or gonococcal infection.
- Ophthalmia neonatorum is a potentially blinding disease; it needs urgent diagnosis.
- Chlamydia is the most common cause of bacterial neonatal conjunctivitis in England. Although it is often harmless, 10%–20% of infants experience chlamydial pneumonia, which is a serious disease. Therefore, infants should receive topical as well as systemic antibiotics.
- Bilateral redness of the eyes may suggest viral or allergic conjunctivitis, while unilateral redness often suggests FB, which can be detected by everting the upper lid to check for concealed FB.
- Pain is not usually caused by conjunctivitis, but rather by uveitis, keratitis, glaucoma or scleritis.
- EKC is highly infectious, caused by adenovirus type 8. Hygienic measures, e.g. hand washing, are essential to prevent spread of the disease.
- A child with red eyes and impaired vision is unlikely to have conjunctivitis. Keratitis is more likely. Ask whether there is a 'gritty sensation', which occurs with keratitis.
- Steroids should never be prescribed for red eyes unless herpes infection is excluded. If diagnosis is not clear, referral to an ophthalmologist is indicated.
- Orbital cellulitis presents as red and swollen eye and must be differentiated from rhabdomyosarcoma, which is a very aggressive malignancy of embryonic muscle tissue within the orbit. The tumour is often curable with radiation and radiotherapy.

FURTHER READING

Chawla R, Kellner JD, Astle W. Acute infectious conjunctivitis in children. *Paediatr Child Health* 2001;6(6):329–335.

Eye   105

ACUTE AND TRANSIENT LOSS OF VISION

Clinical Overview

Visual loss may be acute or gradual, temporary or permanent. Acute visual loss is a frightening experience not only for children and their parents but also for clinicians. Conditions causing acute visual loss in paediatrics are collectively uncommon (incidence estimated to be 2–5 cases per 10,000 births). It is due to either abnormalities within the ocular structure (cornea, lens, vitreous and retina) or neural visual pathways in the central nervous system (optic nerve, chiasm and cortical area). Visual loss within the eyes is easy to detect, e.g. corneal opacity, cataract or optic atrophy. Most causes of cortical visual loss occur in children with neurodisability such as asphyxia at birth, in association with seizures, spasticity or hypotonia. Rarely cortical visual loss occurs as an isolated neurological phenomenon. This section discusses acute and transient visual loss only.

Possible Diagnoses

Infants	Children
Common	
Eye injury (birth trauma)	Migraine
Birth asphyxia (hypoxic-ischaemic)	Uveitis
Hypoperfusion (anaemia, hypotension)	Infection (e.g. trachoma, meningitis, keratitis)
Thrombosis (e.g. polycythaemia)	Thromboembolic phenomenon
Drugs (e.g. gentamicin)	Raised intracranial pressure (ICP) (tumour, pseudotumour cerebri)
Rare	
	Trauma (e.g. intracranial haemorrhage, stroke)
Toxoplasmosis, rubella, cytomegalovirus and herpes (TORCH) infection	Occipital lobe seizures
HIV infection	Amaurosis fugax
Retinal detachment	Macular degeneration
Congenital varicella	Optic neuritis
	Acute glaucoma
	HIV infection
	Retinal migraine, arterial or venous occlusion
	Conversion symptom (hysteria)
	Cortical blindness
	Familial transient visual loss
	Postprandial transient visual loss
	Unexplained

Differential Diagnosis at a Glance

	Migraine	Uveitis	Infection	Thromboembolic	Raised ICP
Sudden onset	Yes	Possible	Yes	Yes	Possible
Monocular	No	Yes	Possible	Yes	No
With headache	Yes	Possible	Possible	Possible	Yes
Recurrence	Yes	Possible	No	Possible	No
Severe vision loss	No	No	Possible	Possible	No

Recommended Investigations

**   TORCH screening test (polymerase chain reaction and serological tests for cytomegalovirus, herpes simplex virus, rubella virus)

*** HIV DNA detected by polymerase chain reaction

*** Orbital ultrasonography and computed tomography (CT) scan of the eye and head for suspected tumour

*** Electroencephalogram (EEG) for cases with seizures

**   Electroretinography for retinal causes of visual loss

Top Tips

- Eye examination is an essential part of neonatal examination, including using an ophthalmoscope at a distance of 20–25 cm to look for the red reflex. Fundoscopy is usually unnecessary.
- In ophthalmology, more than in any other specialty, observation is the most important technique to detect abnormalities. Get the child interested in visual toys and games such as a bright red object or the light source of a torch.
- Although children with eye problems are often referred to an ophthalmologist, clinicians should be able to perform certain eye examinations. These include examination of the visual fields (looking for wiggling fingers), cornea light reflex, cover tests and fundoscopy. Visual acuity is tested by the child's ability to fixate on and follow an object (such as a brightly coloured toy).
- The most common cause for transient visual loss in children occurs during a visual aura of a classic migraine. Aura is defined by the International Headache Society as a recurrent disorder that develops over 5–29 minutes and lasts for less than 1 hour.
- Transient monocular visual loss lasting 1–5 minutes is usually referred to as amaurosis fugax resulting from cerebral ischaemia (seizure, stroke). While migraine aura may present with flashes of light (photopsia), amaurosis fugax presents as blackout of vision or a curtain across the vision.

Red Flags

- Be aware that a child with leukocoria, a white pupil, has a major clinical implication: the likely cause is either retinoblastoma or cataract. Untreated or with delayed treatment, the retinoblastoma will lead to death and cataract to permanent vision loss.
- Be aware of the long-term use of steroids that can cause cataract and glaucoma.
- Conditions causing sudden loss of vision: migraine or amaurosis fugax; thromboembolic events may occur in predisposed conditions such as polycythaemia, sickle-cell anaemia, and homocystinuria.
- Be aware that migraine occurring within 1 hour of visual loss is typical for retinal migraine.
- Any red eyes should not be treated with topical steroids before herpes keratitis is excluded.
- Occipital seizures (such as benign partial epilepsy with occipital paroxysm) are not rare; visual symptoms are prominent and include amaurosis, multi-coloured illusions or hallucinations and eye deviation, followed by hemiclonic seizures or automatisms. EEG is usually diagnostic.
- While papilloedema is a cardinal sign of increased ICP, in infants, separation of the cranial sutures and bulging of the anterior fontanelle decompress the ICP; papilloedema is not seen.

FURTHER READING

Smith JA, Mackensen F, Sen HN et al. Epidemiology and course of disease in childhood uveitis. *Ophthalmology* 2009;116(8):1544–1551.

DOUBLE VISION (DIPLOPIA)

Clinical Overview

Diplopia – simultaneous perception of two images of a single object – is less common in children than in adults because of the lower incidence of strokes and other intracranial lesions. The most common cause of diplopia in children is misalignment of the visual axes, occurring particularly in disorders affecting the cranial nerves (third, fourth and sixth) innervating the six ocular muscles. Other causes involve mechanical interference with ocular motion or disorder of neuromuscular transmission. Diplopia is either binocular (true diplopia) or monocular. The latter is caused by abnormality in the cornea (e.g. severe astigmatism, irregular curvature), in the lens (e.g. cataract, dislocated lens) or in the vitreous humour (e.g. vitreous cysts). Diplopia is often the first manifestation of many systemic muscular or neurologic disorders, some of a serious nature, so prompt evaluation is usually required. A detailed history and examination will make it possible to determine which muscles and ocular nerves are affected and what is the likely cause. Although diplopia does occur in infants, they do not usually present with diplopia and therefore the causes in infants are not included in this section.

Possible Diagnoses

Children

Common

Physiological
Strabismus (particularly paralytic)
Post-surgery for refractive errors
Raised ICP
Myasthenia gravis (MG)

Rare

Trauma
Drugs (e.g. anti-epileptics)
Ophthalmoplegic migraine
Thyroid ophthalmopathy
Retinoblastoma
Conversion symptom (hysteria)
Basilar artery migraine
Möbius syndrome
Stroke
Sarcoidosis

Differential Diagnosis at a Glance

	Physiological	Strabismus	Post-Surgery	ICP	Myasthenia
Normal eyes	Yes	No	No	No	Yes
Associated ptosis	No	No	Possible	Possible	Yes
With headache/vomiting	No	No	No	Yes	No
Associated squint	No	Yes	Possible	Possible	No
The only symptom	Yes	No	No	No	Possible

Recommended Investigations

  **   Urine and plasma amino acid analysis
  *** IV injection of short-acting edrophonium (Tensilon) to reverse the symptoms of MG
  *** Anti-acetylcholine antibodies in plasma for suspected MG
  *** Thyroid function tests for suspected cases of hyperthyroidism
  *** A chest X-ray for suggested case of sarcoidosis to show bilateral hilar lymphadenopathy
  *** Cranial MRI may show tumour, area of infarction or even arterial aneurysm
  *** Electromyogram (EMG) may be diagnostic in cases of MG

Top Tips

- Physiological diplopia is a common and normal phenomenon in which objects not within the area of fixation (in the front or behind) are seen as double.
- Monocular ptosis is easily diagnosed. If diplopia persists with one eye occluded, the patient has monocular diplopia, the causes of which are ophthalmological, usually refractory error. Binocular diplopia resolves when one eye is occluded, usually caused by misalignment of the visual axes.
- The most common cause of diplopia is strabismus. However, the brain of a young child learns how to suppress the image of the weaker, misaligned eye. Therefore, diplopia is usually not the presenting complaint in young age.
- Differentiating monocular from binocular diplopia is simple: covering each eye will correct diplopia in binocular while diplopia persists in the monocular of the affected eye.
- Ophthalmoplegic migraine presents as third-nerve palsy ipsilateral to the hemicranial headache due to vasoconstriction during the attack to this nerve.
- Diplopia may be the first complaint in children with dislocated lens, occurring in Marfan's syndrome (excessive height, dilated aortic route) or homocystinuria (malar flush, neurodisability, thromboembolic events).

Red Flags

- Any diplopia warrants prompt evaluation; it may signal a serious intracranial disease.
- Although diplopia is a common symptom in posterior fossa tumour, children rarely complain of it, as they are able to suppress the image of the affected eye. Instead, head tilting or turning may occur in an attempt to align the two images.
- Beware that fourth-nerve palsy typically presents with head tilting opposite to the affected eye, while the head turns toward the affected eye in sixth-nerve palsy.
- Basilar arterial migraine (diplopia, vertigo, ataxia and headache) should be differentiated from intracranial tumour. An urgent CT scan or MRI is needed, particularly if it is the first episode.
- Diplopia and ptosis may be due to third-nerve palsy or Horner's syndrome. Small pupil and reduced sweating on the affected side will help to differentiate both conditions.
- Remember that the sixth cranial nerve has a long intracranial course so it is susceptible to the effects of raised ICP.
- Adolescents with hysteria may present with diplopia; this diagnosis should be one of exclusion.

FURTHER READING

Danchaivijitr C, Kennard C. Diplopia and eye movement disorders. *J Neurol Neurosurg Psychiatry* 2004;75(Suppl 4):24–31.

EYELID DISORDERS AND PTOSIS

Clinical Overview

Eyelid disorders are exceedingly common in children and range from benign and self-resolving to serious malignant or metastatic processes. Although the majority of these disorders are dealt with by ophthalmologists, this section only stresses those disorders that are important to clinicians in relation to associated systemic diseases. Blepharoptosis, commonly abbreviated as ptosis, is defined as an abnormally low-lying upper eyelid margin on gaze. Eyelid elevation is primarily provided by levator palpebrae superioris muscle with its function to lift the upper eyelid by 5 mm or greater. Congenital ptosis is usually caused by levator muscle dysgenesis. An acquired ptosis may be due to third-nerve palsy, caused by MG, myotonic dystrophy, botulism or Horner's syndrome. Therefore, the diagnosis of any eyelid abnormality requires thorough systemic examination and investigations to exclude systemic diseases.

Possible Diagnoses

Infants	Children
Common	
Coloboma	Congenital ptosis
Congenital ptosis	Acquired ptosis
Congenital ectropion	Acquired Horner's syndrome (with miosis, anhidrosis)
Tumour (haemangioma, dermoid cyst)	Tumour/cyst (e.g. haemangioma, cyst, mechanical ptosis)
Congenital Horner's syndrome	Acute blepharitis
Rare	
Congenital core myopathy	
Congenital entropion	Meibomian cyst
Congenital muscular dystrophy	Chalazion (inflammation of the meibomian cyst)
Congenital MG	Myasthenia gravis (MG)
	Myotonic muscular dystrophy (Steinert's disease)
	Muscular dystrophy (facioscapulohumeral type)
	Blepharophimosis
	Marcus Gunn jaw-winking phenomenon
	Sparse or absent eyebrows (ectodermal dysplasia)
	Lash abnormalities
	Eyebrow abnormalities
	Mitochondrial disorders

Differential Diagnosis at a Glance

	Congenital Ptosis	Acquired Ptosis	Horner's Syndrome	Tumour	Acute Blepharitis
Bilateral	Possible	Possible	Possible	No	Possible
The only finding	Yes	No	No	No	Possible
Inflammatory changes	No	No	No	Possible	Yes
Progressive	No	Possible	Possible	Yes	Possible
Amblyopia	No	Possible	Possible	Possible	No

Recommended Investigations

   *** Creatine phosphokinase in blood for muscular diseases

   *** Anti-acetylcholine and muscle-specific kinase (MUSK) antibodies in plasma for suspected MG

   *** A chest X-ray in cases of MG for evidence of enlarged thymus and thymoma

   ** ECG for cases of muscular dystrophy and myopathies

   *** CT scan of the anterior mediastinum to assess the thymus (thymoma)

   *** EMG for suspected cases of MG or myotonic dystrophy

   *** If MG is suspected, consider referral for neostigmine or edrophonium testing

Top Tips

- When children raise the eyebrows or lift the chin to look around, this may be because of ptosis in an attempt to maintain binocular vision.
- Telecanthus (increased width between the medial canthi) and epicanthus inversus (epicanthic folds originating from the lower lid) can cause ptosis. The latter may be inherited as autosomal dominant; affected females are often infertile.
- Children with ptosis should be referred for ophthalmic opinion and surgery if they have abnormal head posture, amblyopia and abnormal visual field, and if it is cosmetically unacceptable.
- In Marcus Gunn jaw-winking (5% of all cases with ptosis), the upper lid rises as the jaw opens. This is caused by synkinesis between the third and fifth cranial nerves.
- Eyebrow abnormalities include sparse or absent eyebrows (e.g. alopecia, ectodermal dysplasia) and eyebrows joining together medially (Waardenburg or Cornelia de Lange syndrome).

Red Flags

- Ptosis can be due to congenital Horner's syndrome that is associated with vertebral anomalies. The acquired type may be the first presentation of mediastinal tumour such as neuroblastoma.
- There is a high incidence of amblyopia in ptosis due to occlusive stimulus deprivation.
- Beware that entropion (inward-turning of the lid margin and lashes, trichiasis) often presents with irritability and can cause corneal damage. Urgent consultation with an ophthalmologist is required. Larsen syndrome (entropion, multiple joint dislocations, cleft palate and neurodisability) has to be excluded.
- Patients with ectropion (outward-turning of the lid margin) are at risk of exposure keratopathy, overflow of tears and conjunctivitis. This may occur in association with facial palsy resulting from weakness of the orbicularis muscle. Again, urgent ophthalmic consultation is required.
- When the edrophonium (Tensilon) test is carried out to confirm MG, the facility for cardiopulmonary resuscitation must be available. Prior to the test, the ptosis and strabismus are measured.

FURTHER READING

Jubbal KT, Kania K, Brawn TL et al. Pediatric blepharoptosis. *Semin Plast Surg* 2017;31(1):58–64.

PROPTOSIS (EXOPHTHALMOS)

Clinical Overview

Proptosis, exophthalmos or protrusion of the eyes, is a forward displacement of the eye, which may be caused by a congenital shallow orbit (craniofacial malformation such as oxycephaly, Crouzon syndrome), trauma (orbital haemorrhage), inflammation (orbital cellulitis, abscess), vascular diseases (e.g. haemangioma, cavernous sinus thrombosis), central nervous system anomaly (encephalocele), endocrine disorder (e.g. Graves' disease) and neoplasms (optic glioma, meningioma, metastatic neuroblastoma). Children with neurofibromatosis type 1 (NF-1) are at high risk of developing optic glioma and meningioma. The condition provides a diagnostic dilemma.

Possible Diagnoses

Infants	Children
Common	
Orbital capillary haemangioma	Capillary haemangioma
Lymphangioma	Orbital cellulitis
Lacrimal gland cyst/tumour	Shallow orbit (e.g. Crouzon syndrome)
Orbital teratoma	Tumour (optic nerve glioma, meningioma)
Metastatic neuroblastoma	Graves' disease (thyroid orbitopathy)
Rare	
Plexiform neurofibroma	Deep dermoid cyst
Congenital orbital varices	Plexiform neurofibroma
Orbital encephalocele	Trauma (orbital haemorrhage)
Neonatal Graves' disease	Histiocytosis X
	Sarcoidosis
	Lymphangioma
	Neuroblastoma
	Non-specific orbital inflammatory syndrome
	Fibrous dysplasia
	Orbital encephalocele
	Wegener's granulomatosis
	Juvenile xanthogranuloma

Differential Diagnosis at a Glance

	Capillary Haemangioma	Orbital Cellulitis	Shallow Orbit	Tumour	Graves' Disease
Acute onset	No	Yes	No	Possible	No
Unilateral	Yes	Yes	No	Yes	No
Red/tender	No	Yes	No	Possible	No
Lid retraction	No	Possible	No	Possible	Yes
Associated headache/diplopia	No	Possible	No	Possible	Possible

Recommended Investigations

** FBC: leukocytosis suggests bacterial inflammation

*** Thyroid function tests for suspected hyperthyroidism

*** Tumour markers in urine (vanillylmandelic acid and homovanillic acid): elevated in neuroblastoma in 95%
* Skull X-ray for cranial tumour
*** Renal ultrasound scan for metastatic neuroblastoma
*** CT scan (most useful) for any suspected cranial tumour
** Aspiration cytology and biopsy occasionally required

Top Tips

- Orbital capillary haemangioma is the most common orbital tumour in children, more often affecting the upper lid. Remember that the tumour has rapid growth during the first 6 months of life and regresses spontaneously when the child reaches 4–6 years of age.
- A clinician faced with a child with proptosis should be able to undertake ophthalmic examination, including assessment of visual acuity, ocular muscle movement, proptosis, pupillary size and reaction to light, fundi and systemic examination.
- Optic gliomas are common with NF-1 (15%); they are usually benign and asymptomatic and commonly present with visual disturbance. Unilateral glioma typically presents with afferent pupillary defect; a light source on the affected eye produces pupil dilatation (instead of constriction), while the unaffected eye produces bilateral pupil constriction.
- Proptosis caused by Graves' disease may occur in older children. Optic neuropathy, corneal problems and extraocular muscular involvement are far less common in children than in adults. Lid oedema, lag and retraction are common.
- Neuroblastoma, the most common solid tumour of childhood, metastasises frequently into the orbit. The tumour may arise from the adrenals, cervical sympathetic chain or mediastinum.

Red Flags

- A proptotic eye not adequately protected by the lids is at risk of keratopathy, strabismus, diplopia, optic nerve atrophy and decreased visual acuity. Urgent management is required.
- Be aware that orbital cellulitis, often caused by paranasal sinusitis, first manifests as a red swelling of the lid. Prompt treatment with IV antibiotics at this stage dramatically improves the outcome.
- Orbital cellulitis must be recognised and treated promptly before serious complications occur, including extension of the infection into the cranial cavity causing meningitis, cavernous sinus thrombosis, and epidural, subdural, or brain abscess. Admission to hospital is urgently required.
- Be aware that a rapidly progressive swelling may suggest a malignant tumour such as rhabdomyosarcoma, metastatic neuroblastoma or Ewing's sarcoma.
- In a child who presents with Horner's syndrome with or without orbital ecchymoses, neuroblastoma has to be excluded.

FURTHER READING

Chan W, Wong GWK, Fan DSP et al. Ophthalmopathy in children with Graves' disease. *Br J Ophthalmol* 2002;86(7):740–742.

SQUINT (STRABISMUS)

Clinical Overview

Strabismus – misalignment of the eyes – is a common ophthalmic problem, affecting 4%–5% of children younger than 6 years of age (Figure 9.2). It is associated with a significant negative impact on quality of life. Early detection and repair prevent visual and psychosocial dysfunction. Strabismus is diagnosed clinically, which involves examination of the corneal light reflex and cover test. It may be transient or constant, and manifest or latent. Because of different causes and treatments, it is important to divide strabismus into non-paralytic and paralytic. Non-paralytic strabismus includes inward deviation of the eyes (esophorias, commonly known as convergent or inward or crossed eyes), outward deviation of the eyes (known as exophorias, or divergent strabismus) and hyperdeviation (upward) and hypodeviation (downward) of an eye. Paralytic strabismus involves palsy of the third, fourth or sixth cranial nerve. Strabismus may be a congenital (or better termed *infantile*, as this allows inclusion of cases of strabismus that develop within the first few months of life) or an acquired form. One of the most important and serious causes of the acquired form of strabismus is retinoblastoma.

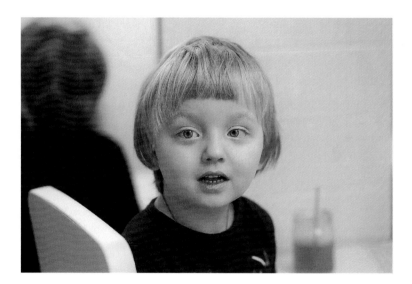

FIGURE 9.2   Squint.

Possible Diagnoses

Infants	Children
Common	
Pseudo-strabismus	Pseudo-strabismus
Congenital (infantile)	Congenital (infantile) non-paralytic strabismus
Intermittent strabismus	Paralytic strabismus
Paralytic strabismus	Accommodation strabismus
Latent strabismus	Latent strabismus

(Continued)

(Continued)

Infants	Children
Rare	
Möbius syndrome	Migraine ophthalmoplegia
Parinaud's syndrome	Möbius syndrome (congenital bilateral facial weakness)
Duane syndrome	Duane syndrome (congenital impaired eye motility)
Brown's syndrome	Parinaud's syndrome (congenital weakness in vertical gaze)
	Brown's syndrome (impaired elevation of the eye on adduction)

Differential Diagnosis at a Glance

	Pseudo-Strabismus	Congenital Squint	Paralytic Squint	Accommodation Strabismus	Latest Strabismus
Normal corneal reflex	Yes	No	Yes	Yes	Possible
Present younger than 6 months	Yes	Yes	Possible	No	Possible
Easily detectable on examination	Yes	Possible	Yes	Possible	Possible
Associated diplopia	No	Possible	Yes	No	No
Detectable by cover test	No	Yes	No	No	Yes

Recommended Investigations

*** Corneal light reflex for children who are not cooperative (under the age of 3 years)
*** Cover test for children who are cooperative
*** Orbital ultrasonography or CT scan for paralytic strabismus or retinoblastoma

Top Tips

• Pseudo-strabismus, a common cause of referral to an ophthalmologist, is caused by epicanthic folds or broad flat nasal bridge. The normal alignment is shown by the normal corneal light reflexes.
• Children with a high risk of developing strabismus, who need close surveillance, include those with a family history of strabismus, prematurity, congenital ptosis or cataract.
• The conventional method of eye patching in strabismus is associated with low compliance, social stigma and stress. New treatments include liquid crystal display occlusion glasses, and botulinum injections to the extraocular muscle (the latter method has acceptable safety margins).
• An eye deviation that is present only when binocular vision is interrupted (by occlusion of one eye) is termed *latent*, while manifest deviation is present under binocular viewing of both eyes.
• Corneal light reflex is the most rapid and easily performed test to diagnose strabismus, particularly in children who are uncooperative.
• Patients with accommodation strabismus (crossed eye) are typically farsighted (hyperopic).
• Up to the age of 6 months, intermittent strabismus is a normal developmental milestone, occurring particularly as outward deviation in about two-thirds of neonates. After the age of 6 months, it is usually asymptomatic due to a well-developed suppression mechanism.

Red Flags

- Strabismus should never be ignored; it is never outgrown.
- In a child with any ocular disorder, including squints, assessment of the visual acuity is essential.
- Remember that the corneal light reflex is normal in paralytic strabismus.
- Untreated amblyopia (reduced visual acuity) results in permanent vision impairment.
- Be aware that children with intermittent strabismus may present with excessive rubbing of the eyes and sensitivity to the sunlight.
- Be aware that a fourth cranial nerve palsy causes a contralateral head tilt, i.e. a head tilt to the right caused by left-sided palsy, and vice versa. Conversely, a sixth cranial nerve palsy causes head turning towards the same side of the palsy. These maneuvers diminish the associated diplopia.
- Retinoblastoma is most curable if diagnosed early; death is inevitable if untreated.
- Retinoblastoma, with an incidence of one in 20,000 births, is the most important cause of acquired strabismus. The tumour also presents with unilateral or bilateral leukocoria (a white pupil), orbital inflammation and/or a red eye reflex (cat eye).

FURTHER READING

Solebo AL, Austin A, Theodorou M et al. Botulinum toxin chemodenervation for childhood strabismus in England: National and local patterns of practice. *PLOS ONE* 2018;13(6):e0199074.

10 URINARY

BEDWETTING (NOCTURNAL ENURESIS)

Clinical Overview

Bedwetting (nocturnal enuresis [NE]) may present in isolation (monosymptomatic enuresis [MSE]) or in association with daytime incontinence; urge, hesitancy, and straining symptoms; postvoid dribbling; or dysfunctional voiding (non-monosymptomatic enuresis [NMSE]). NE is defined as the involuntary voiding of urine during sleep at least three times a week for at least 3 months in a child 5 years or older. It is the most common chronic childhood complaint affecting over half a million children in the United Kingdom. The incidence of NE at the age of 5 years is about 10%; at the age of 10 years, it is around 5%; and 1%–2% of children continue with bedwetting after puberty. About 15% of children are spontaneously cured annually. NE is divided into primary nocturnal enuresis (PNE) (continue to wet beyond the age of 5 years), affecting 80% of children, and secondary nocturnal enuresis (SNE) (after a previous dry period greater than 6 months) in 20% of children. Causes of PNE include genetic (on chromosomes 12 and 13), delayed maturation, sleep disorders and antidiuretic hormone (ADH) deficiency. Causes of SNE include urinary tract infection (UTI), emotional stress, type 1 diabetes (T1D), child abuse, diabetes insipidus (DI), obstructive sleep apnoea (OSA) and seizure.

Possible Diagnoses

Infants	Children
Common	
	PNE (mostly genetic)
	SNE
	Compulsive fluid drinking
	T1D
	Developmental delay
Rare	
	Renal tubular acidosis/necrosis
	Sickle-cell anaemia (SCA)
	DI
	Bladder neck obstruction
	Congestive cardiac failure
	Chronic renal failure
	Nocturnal seizures

Differential Diagnosis at a Glance

	PNE	SNE	Compulsive Drinking	T1D	Developmental Delay
Positive family history	Yes	Possible	No	Possible	No
Psychogenic	No	Yes	Possible	No	No
Associated polydipsia	No	No	Yes	Yes	Possible
Polyuria	No	No	Yes	Yes	No
Short enuresis history	No	Possible	No	Yes	No

Recommended Investigations

*** Urinalysis and culture for infection, and glycosuria (T1D)

*** Blood glucose, acid-base analysis, urea and electrolytes (U&E), if clinically indicated

*** Renal ultrasound scan in NMSE for anatomy and pre- and postvoid urine residual estimates

*** Consider an overnight EEG or polysomnography if nocturnal seizures or sleep disorder is suspected

Top Tips

- Examination should include the perianal area for excoriation due to itching (may suggest threadworms), the vulva, lumbosacral and lower limbs, and the abdomen for distended bladder.
- Clear urine correlates well with absence of bacteria. Dipstick testing suggests UTI, T1D, renal tubular acidosis (glycosuria without hyperglycaemia) and low specific gravity in DI.
- Reassuring the child (and parents) that there is strong evidence that he/she will be dry in the future is often omitted but very helpful; removing any punishment methods at home is important.
- UTI in children with MSE occurs in about 1%. Despite this, urinalysis is essential at the child's initial visit. UTI is found in around 50% in NMSE, and therefore urinalysis is an essential test.
- Functional bladder capacity (FBC) is defined by the following formula: Age of the child $\times 30 + 30$. Low FBC is frequently associated with NE. Measuring the FBC (first void in the morning) is important. Increased water intake and frequent urination during the daytime improve FBC and NE.
- Nocturia, defined as an amount of urine passed at night that exceeds the FBC, is measured by weighing the bed sheet at night and in the morning after wetting. Alternatively, signs such as excessive urine passed (soaking wet), early wetting (in the first 2 hours of sleep), multiple wetting at night and low specific gravity all suggest nocturia.
- A large proportion of children with NE have nocturia. Treatment with desmopressin should primarily be offered for children with evidence of excessive urine output at night.

Red Flags

- Strong association exists between OSA and NE. Adenoid and/or tonsillar hypertrophy should be excluded. Significant reduction of NE is achieved with surgical repair of the obstruction.
- Remember that although parents commonly lift a child with NE, this should be discouraged as it may encourage the child to wet while asleep during the lifting.
- Persistent dysfunctional void may lead to non-neurogenic neurogenic bladder, which is characterised by failure of the external sphincter to relax during voiding. Children may end with trabeculated bladder, hydronephrosis and renal failure.
- Bedwetting may be a warning sign of physical and/or sexual abuse. If physical examination suspects child abuse, have the child examined by a professional specialised in child abuse.

FURTHER READING

National Institute for Clinical Excellence (NICE). Nocturnal enuresis: The management of bedwetting in children and young people. *BMJ* 2010;341. doi.org/10.1136/bmj.c5399. https://www.org.uk/guidance/cg111
Sinha R, Raut S. Management of nocturnal enuresis-myths and facts. *World J Nephrol* 2016;6(4):328–338.

BLOOD IN URINE (HAEMATURIA)

Clinical Overview

Gross haematuria indicates blood is seen with naked eyes. Microscopic haematuria is more common (incidence 1%–2% of school-age children) and is defined as >5 RBC/HPF (red blood cells per high-power field) in the urine sediment of centrifuged freshly voided urine. In contrast to gross haematuria, the majority of patients (about 80%) with microhaematuria have no clinically identifiable cause for the haematuria. The haematuria of glomerular disease is usually uniformly red, without clots or pain. An exception is Henoch–Schönlein purpura (HSP), which is associated with abdominal pain. Causes of painful haematuria include urolithiasis, UTI or renal tumour. When a child presents with blood in urine, doctors should determine that it is actually haematuria. Red urine may be due to drugs (e.g. rifampicin, nitrofurantoin), metabolic causes (e.g. porphyrins, methaemoglobin), pigments (e.g. haemoglobin, myoglobin) and food (e.g. beets, blackberries). In these conditions, urinalysis will be negative for blood.

Possible Diagnoses

Infants	Children
Common	
Asphyxia (hypoxic-ischaemic encephalopathy)	IgA nephropathy
Renal vein thrombosis (cross haematuria)	Poststreptococcal glomerulonephritis (PSGN)
Blood coagulopathy	HSP
Drugs	UTI
Infection (sepsis)	Coagulopathies (e.g. thrombocytopenia)
Obstructive uropathy	
Rare	
Haemorrhagic disease of the newborn (HDN)	Renal stones
Trauma	Vascular (e.g. renal vein thrombosis, SCA)
Renal artery/vein thrombosis	Haemolytic uraemic syndrome (HUS)
Cortical and medullary necrosis	Systemic lupus erythematosus (SLE)
Nephrocalcinosis	Idiopathic haematuria
Polycystic kidney disease	Tumour (e.g. nephroblastoma, bladder hamartoma)
Nephrocalcinosis	Alport syndrome
Tumour (e.g. nephroblastoma)	Polycystic kidneys
	Goodpasture syndrome (pulmonary haemorrhage)
	Drugs
	Hypercalciuria
	Haemorrhagic cystitis (cyclophosphamide)
	High-intensity exercise
	Wegener's granulomatosis (with polyangiitis)
	Nutcracker syndrome (compressed left renal vein)
	Urethral or bladder foreign body

Differential Diagnosis at a Glance

	UTI	PSGN	IgA	HSP	Coagulopathy
Abdominal pain	Possible	No	No	Yes	Possible
With proteinuria	Possible	Yes	Yes	Yes	No
RBCs casts	No	Yes	Yes	Yes	No
Gross haematuria	Possible	Yes	Yes	Yes	Possible
Recurrent	Possible	No	Yes	No	Possible

Recommended Investigations

*** Urine: RBCs and proteinuria suggest renal disease; RBCs casts indicate glomerulonephritis

*** 24-hour urine collection for calcium excretion (abnormal if >4 mg/kg)

*** FBC: anaemia in HUS, haemolytic anaemia, chronic renal disease; leucopenia in SLE, thrombocytopenia in SLE; reticulocytosis in haemolytic anaemia

*** High antistreptolysin titer (or better streptozyme if available) suggests PSGN

*** U&E: increased creatinine and urea in HUS, chronic renal failure; calcium to rule out hypercalcaemia

** Complement levels: low but recover in 6–8 weeks in PSGN; persistent in proliferative nephritis

** Auto-antibodies (ANF, anti-double-stranded DNA antibody for immune-mediated nephritis)

*** Renal ultrasound scan: detects hydronephrosis, calculus, tumour and calcification

*** Cystoscopy for bladder source of bleeding, e.g. haemangiomas, or from a lesion in the ureter

*** In tropics search for *Schistosoma haematobium* eggs in urine and faeces

Top Tips

- Nephrocalcinosis is not uncommon in premature babies and can be seen in up to 40%. Risk factors include the use of loop diuretics, metabolic acidosis and renal tubular acidosis.
- Isolated microscopic haematuria is common in healthy children and often transient. Persistent microscopic haematuria indicates >5 RBC/HPF at monthly intervals.
- Microscopic haematuria is often idiopathic. The most known cause is hypercalciuria (about 25% of cases) and is confirmed by elevated calcium excretion of >4 mg/kg in 24-hour urine collection. Hypercalcaemic hypercalciuria (e.g. hyperparathyroidism) is confirmed by high serum calcium.
- Proteinuria in association with haematuria is very suggestive of renal origin of the haematuria. Casts, particularly RBCs casts, indicate a diagnosis of glomerulonephritis.
- Gross haematuria in association with mild oedema, hypertension and high creatinine suggests nephritic syndrome, while gross oedema and proteinuria suggest nephrotic syndrome.
- IgA nephropathy is the most common cause of recurrent painless haematuria affecting typically children aged 8–10 years. There is concurrent URTI and proteinuria. Haematuria subsides soon to be followed by microscopic haematuria. Diagnosis by biopsy: mesangial deposits in the glomeruli.
- In PSGN, the most common cause of gross haematuria worldwide, the urine is uniformly red, either brownish-red or dark brown (cola colour), and usually contains RBCs casts. Significant abdominal pain is usually absent, except in cases with HSP.
- In many countries, e.g. Egypt, haematuria is mostly due to *Schistosoma haematobium*. Diagnosis is made by detection of eggs in urine and faeces, or biopsy of the bladder, rectum or liver.

Red Flags

- Common presentation of neonatal renal vein and artery thrombosis is gross haematuria, thrombocytopenia and abdominal mass (in vein thrombosis). Hypertension occurs with arterial thrombosis, and this sign should be searched for by repeated blood pressure measurements.
- When a child presents with melaena with or without haematuria, he/she may have HDN. Diagnosis is supported by the history of exclusively breastfed child and no vitamin K was given.
- Neonatal vaginal discharge due to maternal hormonal withdrawal is often mistaken for haematuria particularly when the blood is mixed with urine. Parents should be reassured.
- The presence of red-brown or pink discolouration on the nappies is often urate crystals. This is a benign condition and improves rapidly with increased fluid intake.
- Haematuria in association with abdominal pain suggests UTI, HSP, renal stone or tumour. An urgent urinalysis is required in addition to ultrasound scan.
- It is wrong to make a diagnosis of UTI based on urine RBCs or protein or both; positive nitrite and white blood cells (WBCs) in the dipstick are more important indicators in suggesting UTI than these two indices.
- Be aware that although UTI is usually caused by bacterial infection, common respiratory virus, e.g. adenovirus, can cause haemorrhagic cystitis, particularly in immunocompromised status.
- While adults and older children with urolithiasis present nearly always with severe flank pain and haematuria, pre-school children usually present with UTI and a less severe degree of flank pain.
- Gross haematuria following an URTI suggests IgA nephropathy. Diagnosis is not established by serum complement or IGA levels but by renal biopsy showing glomerular IgA immune deposits.

FURTHER READING

Joseph C, Gattineni J. Proteinuria and haematuria in the neonate. *Curr Opin Pediatr* 2016;28(2):202–208.
NICE Guideline: UTI in children and young people. 2017. http://guidance.nice.org.uk/CG054

FREQUENT URINATION

Clinical Overview

The term indicates frequent (more than seven a day in school-age children) voids of small amounts of urine, often associated with urgency. In infancy, voiding is physiologically frequent, as often as 15–20 times a day, occurring by reflex bladder contraction mediated by sympathetic nerve system (T10–L2) and parasympathetic nerve system (S2–S4). In older children, bladder control is achieved through gradual bladder enlargement, leading to an increase of bladder capacity, cortical inhibition of the reflex bladder contraction, and the ability to consciously tighten the external sphincter to prevent incontinence. In paediatrics, the most common cause of frequent urination is an overactive bladder (OAB), with or without UTI. OAB is defined as urinary urgency without specific pathogen or metabolic disease. The condition has to be differentiated from polyuria (frequent of large amount of urine) and incontinence (involuntary loss of urine). Female children are more affected than males.

Possible Diagnoses

Infants	Children
Common	
Physiological	UTI, mainly lower
Nappy dermatitis	Vulvovaginitis
Fever	Overactive bladder (detrusor instability)
Diuretics	Pollakiuria and anxiety (daytime frequent urination)
	Developmental delay (including neurogenic bladder)
Rare	
	Drugs (diuretics)
	Urethritis (e.g. Reiter's syndrome)
	Ectopic ureter and fistula
	Vaginal voiding
	Bladder outlet obstruction
	Urethral stricture
	Pregnancy
	Excessive intake of caffeine
	Congenital bladder diverticulum

Differential Diagnosis at a Glance

	Lower UTI	Vulvovaginitis	OAB	Pollakiuria	Developmental Delay
With dysuria	Yes	Yes	Possible	No	Possible
Positive nitrite and WBC	Yes	Possible	Possible	No	No
Reduced FBC	No	No	Yes	Yes	Yes
More in girls	Yes	Yes	Yes	Possible	No
Fever	Possible	No	No	No	No

Recommended Investigations

   *** Urinalysis with urine culture
   *** Renal ultrasound scan with pre- and postvoid residual urine estimate
   *** Urodynamic study for neurogenic bladder

Top Tips

- Evaluation of the bladder function in older children should begin with keeping, for at least 3 consecutive days, a voiding diary that contains data on the hours and volumes of voided urine to establish the frequency and functional bladder capacity.
- Pollakiuria (from the Greek word *pollakis* meaning 'many times') or daytime frequency syndrome of childhood, often occurs as a result of stress-related problems, including anxiety, but without dysuria or systemic disease. There is sudden onset of frequent voiding every 5–10 minutes, in a previously toilet-trained child. It often disappears suddenly in 2–3 months. Typical age of occurrence is 4–6 years.
- Hypercalciuria may be a sign of overactive bladder.
- Dysfunction voiding is a common cause of frequent urination. It is characterised by a void of a smaller than normal amount of urine or a bladder that contracts against a closed sphincter.
- Children with delayed attainment of bladder control and daytime incontinence have increased risk of incontinence in adolescence.

Red Flags

- In the differential diagnosis of frequent urination, the most important aspect is to exclude polyuria. Arrange a urine collection over 12 or 24 hours to establish the diagnosis if necessary.
- Ensure that the frequent voiding is not continuous incontinence; if so this suggests in boys posterior urethral valve obstruction and in girls ectopic ureter.
- Ectopic ureter usually occurs in girls in association with a duplicate collecting system that can be diagnosed by ultrasound scan. Dribbling incontinence is characteristic and should not be missed.
- When physical examination and urinalysis are normal, hypercalciuria with or without urolithiasis is often the cause. A 24-hour urine collection for calcium is diagnostic.
- Vaginal void may occur because of ectopic ureter into the vagina. Labial adhesions are a common cause of continuous urinary incontinence and frequency. Typically, a girl with labial adhesions urinates after she stands up.
- There is a strong link between child abuse (sexual, emotional and physical) and urological symptoms, even years after the abuse has occurred. This link should be kept in mind when a child presents with urinary frequency and urgency symptoms.

FURTHER READING

Heron J, Grzeda M, von Gontard A et al. Trajectories of urinary incontinence in childhood bladder and bowel symptoms in adolescence: Prospective cohort study. *BMJ Open* 2017;7(3):e014238.
NICE Guideline: UTI in children and young people. 2017. http://guidance.nice.org.uk/CG054

INCONTINENCE (DAYTIME OR DIURNAL WETTING)

Clinical Overview

Urinary incontinence (UI) is a common problem presenting at primary care services, often associated with frequent urination, urge symptoms and NE. It indicates involuntary loss of urine during the daytime (diurnal) after the age of 5 years. It can be primary (child has been persistently incontinent) or secondary if the child achieved complete dryness for a period greater than 6 months. Primary incontinence is usually intermittent with variable periods of continence intervals. On rare occasions it has an organic cause: congenital malformation of the ureter, neurogenic bladder that includes congenital spina bifida and sacral agenesis and acquired inflammatory or neoplastic diseases of the nervous system. Secondary incontinence is usually associated with a stressful event, constipation, T1D, and child abuse. The main causes of UI are an overactive bladder leading to urinary urge and holding urine until the last minute by suppressing the need to void, until incontinence happens. Around 20%–40% of children with UI have behavioural problems including attention deficit hyperactivity disorder, anxiety and antisocial behaviour.

Possible Diagnoses

Infants	Children
Common	
Physiological (before 5 years)	Unstable bladder (overactive bladder)
Congenital malformation (e.g. urethra, ureter)	Lower UTI
Meningomyelocele	Neurogenic bladder
Labial adhesions	Giggle incontinence
Rare	
	Chronic renal failure
	Bladder outlet obstruction (e.g. posterior urethral obstruction)
	Ectopic ureter (in girls)
	Sacral agenesis
	Vulvar lichen sclerosis
	Vaginal reflux of urine
	Balanitis xerotica obliterans
	Hinman syndrome
	Lipomeningocele
	DI
	Tethered spinal cord

Differential Diagnosis at a Glance

	Unstable Bladder	Lower UTI	Neurogenic Bladder	Giggle Incontinence	Labial Adhesions
Episodic	No	No	Possible	Yes	No
Frequent urination	Yes	Yes	Possible	No	Yes
Mainly in girls	No	Possible	No	Yes	Yes
Positive nitrite and WBC	Possible	Yes	Possible	No	Possible
Examination confirms diagnosis	No	No	Yes	No	Yes

Recommended Investigations

*** Urinalysis: positive nitrate and leukocytes suggest UTI, culture will confirm the infection; specific gravity of urine >1.005 excludes DI; 24-hour urine collection needed to exclude hypercalciuria

*** Renal ultrasound scan, with pre- and postvoid residual urine estimates

** Urodynamics and lumbosacral evaluation mainly for cases of neurogenic bladder

*** Spine MRI if tethered cord is suspected.

Top Tips

- Diurnal enuresis, or daytime wetting, is involuntary voiding of urine during waking hours. It occurs in 10% of children aged 4–6 years and in 2% of adults.
- Labial fusion is common, affecting about 3% of prepubertal girls. The labia minora fuse, usually distally, allowing a tiny opening proximally. The pocket behind the fused labia acts as a reservoir from which urine is leaking when the girl is standing or playing.
- Hinman's syndrome is a non-neurogenic (spine is normal) voiding dysfunction caused by uncoordinated activity of the detrusor muscle, bladder neck and external sphincter, often leading subsequently to increased intra-vesical pressure and kidney damage.
- In vaginal reflux, girls, particularly obese, who do not open their labia wide enough when voiding, urine may reflux into the vagina, then leak down and wet the knickers as they stand up.
- In boys, posterior urethral valve is the most common cause of UI.
- A girl who voids normally but is incontinent day and night should be considered to have an ectopic ureter with duplex kidney until proven otherwise. While an ectopic ureter in girls usually terminates within the distal third of the vaginal introitus, in boys it usually terminates within the bladder neck or posterior urethra. Therefore boys do not suffer from incontinence caused by ectopic ureter.
- Successful management of incontinence includes dietary means (eliminating caffeine and orange juice), improving bladder capacity by drinking extra water during the daytime, treating constipation and instructing the child to void regularly every 2–3 hours. Anticholinergic drugs are very helpful.

Red Flags

- Remember to ask the radiologist at the request form for renal ultrasound to measure the bladder wall thickness: if greater than 5 mm, it indicates a bladder outlet obstruction such as bladder-sphincter dyssynergia in girls and posterior valve in boys.
- Giggle incontinence occurs in about 5%–10% of girls. The bladder empties completely during laughter or giggling; it can be very embarrassing in public. Urgent management is needed.
- Daytime incontinence is frequently caused or complicated by UTI. Ensure that the urine sample is examined for UTI each time the child attends the clinic.
- When a girl presents with a history of never gaining urinary control and underwear is always wet, she probably has ectopic bladder. Confirm the diagnosis by drying the vaginal introitus and inspect the area every 15 minutes. Re-accumulation of urine is diagnostic.
- Treatment of a child with night and daytime wetting should focus on the daytime problem first. When daytime wetting responds to the treatment, nighttime wetting will improve, not vice versa.

FURTHER READING

Bernard-Bonnin AC. Diurnal enuresis in childhood. *Can Fam Physician* 2000;46:1109–1115.

PAINFUL URINATION (DYSURIA)

Clinical Overview

Painful or burning urination during or immediately after urination, termed *dysuria*, is often accompanied by other urinary symptoms such as frequency, urgency or hesitancy. Although this can sometimes be a sign of UTI, it is more commonly caused by vulvovaginitis, balanitis or urethritis. The majority of causes of dysuria are self-limiting and identified by physical examination with urine or discharge cultures. Children sometimes express itching as dysuria, and this is commonly seen with worm infestation. Children who have persistent dysuria with a normal examination and negative cultures are likely to have either dysfunctional void or hypercalciuria.

Possible Diagnoses

Infants	Children
Common	
Nappy rash (diaper dermatitis)	UTI, mainly lower UTI
Meatal stenosis/ulceration	Vulvovaginitis
Atopic dermatitis	Balanitis
Balanitis	Urethritis/cystitis
Chemical irritation	Sexually transmitted diseases (STDs)
Rare	
Herpes simplex infection (peri-urethral)	Reiter's syndrome (urethritis, arthritis, red eyes)
Varicella (peri-urethral lesions)	Sexual abuse
	Drugs
	Hypercalciuria (dysuria with haematuria)
	Herpes simplex infection
	Labial adhesions
	Pinworms
	Lichen planus/sclerosis
	Stevens-Johnson syndrome
	Urethral foreign body

Differential Diagnosis at a Glance

	UTI	Vulvovaginitis	Balanitis	STD	Urethritis/Cystitis
Most common cause	Yes	Yes	No	No	No
Positive urine culture	Yes	Possible	No	Possible	Possible
Fever	Possible	No	No	No	No
Bacterial infection	Yes	Possible	Possible	Yes	Possible
Discharge	No	Possible	Possible	Yes	Possible

Recommended Investigations

*** Urinalysis is essential for UTI, including culture to confirm UTI
*** Culture of any discharge in girls with vulvovaginitis to exclude infection or STD
*** Larvae or ova of pinworms from discharge of vulvovaginitis
*** Abdominal ultrasound scan for cases with UTI, according to NICE guidelines

Top Tips

- In children with dysuria, history and examination will determine whether any test is necessary.
- Nappy dermatitis is the most common cause of dysuria in infancy. This is expressed as crying or discomfort during urination.
- Meatal stenosis – abnormal narrowing of the urethral opening (meatus) – may be congenital or acquired, e.g. after circumcision. The condition is characterised by upward, deflected urine, dysuria, urgency, and frequency and prolonged urination.
- Vulvar lichen sclerosis is a chronic dermatosis of unknown aetiology (autoimmune) characterised by white patches or plagues affecting the vulva and anus, and causing irritation, dysuria and UI. In males it is known as balanitis xerotica obliterans.
- Urine dipstick testing is very helpful in suggesting or excluding UTI: the presence of positive nitrite with WBC is suggestive but when both are negative UTI is very unlikely.
- In patients with normal examination and negative cultures, dysuria (often associated with microscopic haematuria) can be caused by hypercalciuria. A 24-hour urine collection is indicated.

Red Flags

- A child with meatal stenosis (congenial or acquired) requires urgent attention to avoid potential chronic incomplete bladder emptying with subsequent UTI and kidney damage.
- A child with vulvovaginitis should undergo a careful history to exclude sexual abuse.
- Remember that a foreign body, such as a piece of toilet paper, can be trapped in the vagina and cause discharge and dysuria. Careful area inspection is essential.
- Beware that pruritis can be expressed as dysuria; pinworms, which normally infest the perianal area, may occasionally spread to the vagina.
- In a female patient with dysuria and abdominal pain, pelvic inflammatory disease (PID) must be ruled out. Asymptomatic infections with either *Neisseria gonorrhoeae* or *Chlamydia trachomatis* may lead to the development of PID, which has serious consequences if left untreated.
- A urethral or vaginal discharge in an adolescent is likely caused by an infection with either *N. gonorrhoeae* or *C. trachomatis.*
- Painful micturition is a serious problem for it may cause urine retention with subsequent dilation of the urinary tract system. When herpes simplex causes urethritis, vesicles may be tiny and inapparent; a thorough examination can clench the diagnosis.
- Beware that in older children self-exploratory sexual play and masturbation can cause balanitis or vulvovaginitis, even if the history is negative.

FURTHER READING

NICE Guideline: UTI in children and young people. 2017. http://guidance.nice.org.uk/CG054

POLYURIA (EXCESSIVE URINATION)

Clinical Overview

Kidney has a key role in the body water balance: an increase in plasma osmolality (even less than 1%) or decrease in blood volume stimulates osmo-receptors in the hypothalamus, leading to secretion of the ADH arginine vasopressin (AVP) from the pituitary gland. AVP binds to the type 2 vasopressin (VAP) receptor on the distal tubules and collecting system to increase water re-absorption through the cyclic AMP-mediated pathway. Polyuria is defined as urine output >2 $L/m^2/24$ h resulting from either water or solute diuresis. The most common cause of polyuria is T1D, which is an autoimmune polygenic disease. DI arises if there is no production or release of ADH or the kidney is unresponsive to the ADH due to mutated VAP receptor. Other causes include failure of renal tubular concentration ability (e.g. SCA) and excessive drinking (compulsive drinking). Polyuria must be differentiated from the more common complaint of frequency of a small volume of urine. Accurate measurement of 24-hour intake of fluids and quantity of urine excretion should be performed to establish diagnosis of polyuria. Children with polyuria may present with polydipsia, failure to thrive, dehydration, elevated body temperature (hyperthermia), seizure due to hypernatraemic dehydration and NE.

Possible Diagnoses

Infants	Children
Common	
Post-asphyxia	T1D
Congenital nephrogenic diabetes insipidus (NDI)	Psychogenic polydipsia (compulsive fluid drinking)
Neonatal diabetes	Renal tubular acidosis
Barter's syndrome	DI, cranial
Hypercalcaemia	Metabolic polyuria (potassium deficiency, hypercalcaemia)
Rare	
	Congenital and acquired NDI
	SCA
	Hypercalcaemia
	Polycystic kidney disease
	Chronic renal failure
	Drugs (diuretics, lithium, chlortetracycline)
	Drugs affecting renal tubule
	Renal tubular acidosis (e.g. Fanconi's syndrome)
	Pituitary tumours (craniopharyngioma, histiocytosis X)
	Barter's syndrome
	Post-renal transplant
	Cystic fibrosis–associated diabetes

Differential Diagnosis at a Glance

	T1D	Compulsive	Renal Tubular Acidosis	Cranial DI	Metabolic Polyuria
Weight loss	Yes	No	Yes	Possible	Possible
Short history	Yes	No	No	Possible	Possible
Glycosuria	Yes	No	Yes	No	No
Acidosis	Yes	No	Yes	No	Possible
Hyperglycaemia	Yes	No	No	No	No

Recommended Investigations

*** Urinalysis will confirm glycosuria and ketones in DM; specific gravity: low in DI
*** Blood glucose (BG), to confirm T1D; acid balance and ketones to confirm DKA
*** HbA1c on admission and three monthly for T1D
*** Osmolality of serum and urine; urine-specific gravity
** FBC: anaemia is usually present in chronic renal failure and SCA
*** U&E, high creatinine in chronic renal failure; high Na in polyuria
*** Serum calcium: high in hypercalcaemia
** ADH serum level estimation in DI: low in cranial DI and normal in NDI
*** Cranial MRI for the central causes of DI such as craniopharyngioma
*** Water deprivation test to differentiate between central and NDI

Top Tips

- Although the history and physical examination provide clues to the majority of causes of polyuria, the definite diagnosis is established from biochemical results: blood glucose, osmolality of the urine and serum and U&E.
- It is essential to determine whether the child has frequent, small urination or polyuria (large urine). Mothers are good historians. Observing the child's urination helps to establish a diagnosis.
- Of all polyuria causes, the most common and important is T1D presenting with characteristic symptoms of polyuria, polydipsia, weight loss and high BG (HbA1c $\geq$ 6.5% or fasting BG: 7.0 mmol = 126 mg/dL). The goals of treatment are near normalisation of glucose metabolism (HbA1c < 7.5% = 58.5 mmol), and prevention of acute (hypoglycaemia, ketoacidosis) and long-term complications (retinopathy, neuropathy, nephropathy, high lipids).
- Children with compulsive drinking are easily diagnosed by the long history, absence of weight loss and failure to thrive. Low serum osmolality (<280 mosm/kg) and urine-specific gravity <1.005 establishes the diagnosis. A specific gravity greater than 1.005 excludes DI.
- Compulsive thirst needs to be differentiated from DI (defined as >50 mL/kg body weight/24 h) that has high serum osmolality and low urine osmolality <300 mosm.
- The fourth most important cause of polyuria is renal tubular acidosis. Children may present with dehydration, failure to thrive, anorexia and vomiting. Diagnosis is by finding glycosuria, low serum bicarbonate and potassium and hyperchloraemia.

Red Flags

- Polyuria due to hypercalcaemia or NDI may pass unnoticed and the infant may present in the first few weeks of life with irritability, poor feeding, weight loss, fever and seizure. These can have potentially devastating consequences (e.g. brain damage) if left undiagnosed and untreated.
- Be aware that although NDI occurs virtually only in boys, the female carrier may present with infant polyuria due to impaired urine concentration ability.
- Long-standing polyuria may cause enlarged bladder, mega-ureter and hydronephrosis.
- The water deprivation test is performed to differentiate cranial DI from NDI. The risk of severe dehydration and hypovolaemia is real; therefore, strict control is required.

FURTHER READING

Simmons KM, Michels AW. Type 1 diabetes: A predicable disease. *World J Diabetes* 2015;6(3):380–390.

URINE RETENTION AND FAILURE TO PASS URINE

Clinical Overview

Retention of urine is a frequent presentation in adults (mainly due to benign prostatic hypertrophy) but is relatively infrequent in children. It is defined as inability to void for >12 hours, palpable distended bladder on physical examination or greater than expected volume in bladder in a child without previously known neurological abnormalities, voiding dysfunction, immobility or recent surgery. Healthy neonates are expected to pass urine within 48 hours of life; failure to void after 48 hours is abnormal and requires careful examination and investigation. Neurological control of the bladder consists of a storage phase (stimulated by T10–L2) with sympathetic relaxation of the detrusor muscle and contraction of the urethral sphincter, and a voiding phase where parasympathetic stimulation facilitates detrusor muscle contraction and urethral sphincter relaxation (stimulated by S2–S4).

Possible Diagnoses

Infants	Children
Common	
Shock	
Urethral valve obstruction	Neurological abnormalities
Asphyxia	Dysfunctional voiding (DV)
Dehydration	UTI
Neurogenic bladder	Constipation
Acute renal failure	Drugs (anticholinergic, antidepressants)
Acute tubular necrosis	
Urethral stricture	
Rare	
Imperforate hymen	Imperforate hymen
Acute genital herpes	Local inflammatory (balanitis, labial fusion)
Congestive cardiac failure	Urethral calculus
Bilateral renal agenesis	Foreign body inserted into the urethra
Bilateral renal vein thrombosis	Bladder neck obstruction

Differential Diagnosis at a Glance

	Neurological	Dysfunctional Void	UTI	Constipation	Drugs
Abnormal urinalysis	No	Possible	Yes	Possible	No
Dysuria	No	Possible	Possible	Possible	Possible
Fever	No	No	Possible	No	Possible
Complete retention	No	No	No	Possible	Possible
Examination establishes the cause	Yes	No	No	Yes	No

Recommended Investigations

   *** Urine dipstick: haematuria suggests urinary calculus or bladder tumour
   *** U&E: high creatinine suggests renal failure
   *** Renal ultrasound scan for any structural abnormalities, dilated urethra, bladder and ureter

Top Tips

- A normal neonate has 6–44 mL of urine in the bladder at birth. About 90% of newborns pass urine within 24 hours; the remaining pass urine within 48 hours.
- DV applies to children who habitually contract the urethral sphincter during voiding. DV is associated with constipation, painful local irritation (e.g. vulvitis, balanitis), fear of unclean toilet and urge symptom of urination with attempt to avoid voiding.
- It is important to differentiate between anuria and retention. In the latter the bladder is usually full, but it is empty with anuria. History, radiology and U&E differentiate between these conditions.
- Labial fusion (or adhesions) is a common condition (up to 3% of prepubertal girls have it) of urinary retention; topical oestrogen is indicated. Surgical intervention may be required.

Red Flags

- DV results in bladder outflow obstruction and urine retention, leading to a spectrum of presentations from recurrent lower UTI to significant upper tract pathology and renal failure. Treating the cause of the DV is essential.
- All cases of urethral valve obstruction require admission for evaluation and management. Catheterisation of the bladder should not be attempted before you contact a renal unit as this procedure may destroy the valve and a diagnosis can be missed.
- Anticholinergic drugs used to stabilise the bladder for diurnal incontinence may cause retention, dry mouth and constipation. Parents should be warned about these possible side effects.
- A chronically distended bladder should not be fully drained by catheterization; sudden decompression can cause haematuria and other renal complications. Haematuria can cause clots in the urethra leading to urine retention and bladder distension.

FURTHER READING

Clothier J, Wright AJ. Dysfunctional voiding: The importance of non-invasive urodynamics in diagnosis and treatment. *Pediatr Nephrol* 2018;33(3):381–394.

11 GENITAL

GROIN SWELLING AND PAIN

Clinical Overview

Swelling of the groin in infants and young children is common and usually noticed by the mother while giving the child a bath. Lymphadenopathy and inguinal hernia (IH) are the two most common causes. An important finding in this area is spermatic cord hydrocele, which is a fluid collection along the spermatic cord; it results from abnormal closure of the processus vaginalis and is separated from the testis and epididymis. It has two types: an encysted hydrocele, which does not communicate with the peritoneum, and a communicating hydrocele, where the fluid collection communicates with the peritoneum. Lymphadenopathy is mostly caused by local inflammation such as nappy rash. Groin pain often accompanies groin swelling, is caused by a tear or rupture to any adductor thigh muscles following trauma, and produces sudden sharp pain in the thigh. Other causes of groin pain include transient synovitis (irritable hip), hip avascular necrosis (Perthes' disease) and hip arthritis.

Possible Diagnoses

Infants	Children
Common	
IH	IH
Lymphadenopathy (from nappy rash)	Infectious lymphadenopathy
Hydrocele of spermatic cord	Hydrocele of spermatic cord
Undescended testis	Undescended testis (true undescended)
Testicular feminisation	Femoral hernia
Rare	
	Cancerous lymphadenopathy
	Testicular feminisation
	Lymphangioma
	Epididymal/epidermoid cyst
	Lymphatic malignancy

Differential Diagnosis at a Glance

	IH	Lymphadenitis	Hydrocele Spermatic Cord	Undescended Testis	Femoral Hernia
Pain/tender	No	Yes	No	No	No
Bilateral	Possible	Possible	No	Possible	No
Reducible	Yes	No	No	No	Yes
Palpable testis	Yes	Yes	Yes	No	Yes
Transillumination	Yes	No	Yes	No	Yes

Recommended Investigations

Diagnosis of groin swelling is clinical and investigations are usually not required.

** Full blood count and C-reactive protein are often required in case of lymphadenitis
** Ultrasound scan is useful in differentiating solid mass (lymph node from hydrocele, hernia)
** Further tests (such as biopsy) may be required if the lymphadenopathy suggests malignancy

Top Tips

- Children with cystic fibrosis, undescended testes, connective tissue diseases, contralateral hernia, and prematurity (up to 30% of very low birth infants) have a very high incidence of IH.
- Transillumination demonstrates the presence of fluid: if light shines through, the swelling is cystic; if not, the mass is solid.
- It is important to differentiate between true undescended and retractile (yo-yo) testis. In the retractile testis the scrotum is well developed (while it is hypoplastic in true undescended testis) and the testis can be manipulated down into the normal scrotal position.
- IH is almost always symptomatic, and the only cure is surgery. However, recurrences requiring re-operation occur in 10%–15%, and long-term chronic pain in 10%–12%.
- Remember that although a child has around 600 lymph nodes, only the minority of them can be palpated mainly in the neck, submandibular, axillary and inguinal regions. Generalised lymphadenopathy indicates the involvement of at least two of these sites.
- Following a repair of IH, a contralateral hernia develops in about 30%–40%. The risk rises to 50% if the repair of unilateral hernia is performed within the first year of life.
- A child (often aged 5–6 years) with limping and hip pain is likely to have an irritable hip, which is one of the most frequent causes of hip pain. This condition should be differentiated from septic arthritis.

Red Flags

- In adults, it is a common practise to insert the index finger into the inguinal canal to feel for an impulse while the patient is asked to strain or cough. Do not do that in children: the procedure is painful and rarely yields any useful information.
- Unlike umbilical hernias, IH in children are potentially serious. They require repair as soon as possible. Referral to surgeons is urgent if the child is younger than 6 months of age.
- Risk factors for hernia incarceration include female gender, femoral hernia, and groin hernia.
- An IH that cannot be reduced by manipulation (this occurs in only 5%–10%) is often due to narrow processus vaginalis and not necessarily due to incarceration. This latter complication is associated with marked tenderness, a firm mass and a child who inconsolably cries.
- IH in girls is far less common than in boys. A lump in the inguinal area may contain an ovary or, rarely, a testicle. The latter suggests testicular feminisation, which is confirmed by chromosomal analysis showing 46 XY. There is a high incidence of later malignancy in the gonads; it is therefore routine practice to remove them once the diagnosis is established.
- Beware that stony hard lymph nodes usually suggest malignancy, and may be metastatic.

FURTHER READING

HerniaSurge Group. International guidelines for groin hernia. *Hernia* 2018;22(1):1–165.

PENILE SWELLING

Clinical Overview

Penile anomalies are common in children, causing concern for their parents. When a child presents with a penile problem, the paediatrician has to decide whether the condition is benign, and so parents can be reassured, or whether a prompt referral to a surgeon is needed. Swelling of the penis, often with inflammation and pain, may occur in association with nappy rash or forceful attempt to retract the foreskin. Balanitis (inflammation of the glans) and posthitis (inflammation of the prepuce) are usually caused by Gram-positive organisms such as *Staphylococcus*. Priapism, a persistent unwanted erection unrelated to sexual stimulation, is a relatively frequent complication in children with haematological disorders (e.g. sickle-cell anaemia [SCA], G-6-P-D deficiency), medications or trauma. The oedema of nephrotic syndrome (NS) or Henoch–Schönlein purpura (HSP) accumulates in dependent sites and often causes penile swelling. Practically all cases of penile swelling need immediate medical attention.

Possible Diagnoses

Infants	Children
Common	
Trauma (birth injury, e.g. breach delivery)	Balanitis
Balanitis	Trauma
Congenital adrenal hyperplasia (CAH)	Paraphimosis
Associated with nappy rash	Priapism (e.g. in sickle cell anaemia [SCA])
Penile oedema (idiopathic, generalised oedema)	Penile oedema (e.g. nephrotic syndrome [NS])
Rare	
Congenital NS	Drugs (cocaine, serotonin reuptake inhibitors)
Paraphimosis	Penile torsion
Congenital lymphoedema	Para-urethral cyst
	Congenital or post-infectious lymphoedema
	Tumour (including carcinoma)
	Megalo-urethra
	Epidermal inclusion cyst

Differential Diagnosis at a Glance

	Balanitis	Trauma	Paraphimosis	Priapism	Penile Oedema
Inflammatory changes/redness	Yes	Possible	No	No	No
Pain/tenderness	Yes	Yes	Yes	Yes	No
Associated systemic signs	No	Possible	No	Yes	Possible
Engorgement of glans only	Possible	No	Yes	No	No
History of recurrence	Possible	No	Possible	Possible	No

Recommended Investigations

***   Urine to confirm proteinuria in case of NS
***   Hormonal investigation to exclude CAH, such as plasma 17-hydroxyprogesterone

*** Haemoglobin (Hb), Hb-electrophoresis and peripheral blood film for any non-traumatic priapism
*** Plasma albumin, cholesterol and triglycerides for cases of NS
*** Gram-stained smear and culture in case of urethral discharge

Top Tips

- The foreskin is normally non-retractile and attached to the glans in neonates. It becomes retractile in about 40% of children aged 1 year, in 90% aged 4 years and in 99% aged 15 years.
- Balanitis, the most common cause of penile inflammation, may result from allergy, seborrhoeic dermatitis, insect bites or from any erosion of the skin allowing bacteria (usually staphylococci) to invade. Sexually transmitted disease (STD) should be considered in sexually active adolescents.
- Priapism is usually ischaemic, which is rigid and tender. Non-tender priapism is non-ischaemic.
- Priapism in SCA results from pooling of blood in the corpora cavernosa, causing obstruction to the venous outflow. It usually lasts more than 4 hours.
- A rare condition of penile swelling is penile torsion, usually anti-clockwise rotation of the penis.
- Although SCA is the most common cause of priapism, penile neoplasms, leukaemia (particularly chronic granulocytic leukaemia), cocaine abuse and scorpion bite are other rarer causes.
- Penile manifestations of HSP (also termed immunoglobulin A vasculitis) include penile swelling, priapism, purpuric lesions of the penis and penile thrombosis.
- Immediate management of children with priapism includes ice packs, bed rest, emptying the bladder, oral or IV hydration and analgesics. Morphine may be required.

Red Flags

- Attempts to forcefully retract the foreskin (e.g. for cleansing) are dangerous; this can lead to balanitis or paraphimosis.
- An enlarged penis at birth may be the only clinical manifestation of CAH as some degrees of masculinisation are almost always present at birth. In girls, enlargement of the clitoris and labial fusion dominate the clinical features of CAH at birth.
- Be aware that cases of paraphimosis (a retracted foreskin behind the corona glandis that cannot be returned) require immediate attention if ischaemia of the glans is to be prevented. Firm manual compression, with eutectic mixture of local anaesthetics cream and gauze, will usually reduce the constriction.
- Parents of children with SCA should be told to seek medical assistance if their child develops priapism. They should seek immediate medical assistance to prevent ischaemia, erectile dysfunction and impotence in the future.
- Be aware that penile swelling may be the initial sign of NS; check protein in the urine.
- Genital injury in boys caused by physical or sexual abuse is often unrecognised. Any unexplained penile burn, bruising, incised wound and laceration should raise suspicions of child abuse.

FURTHER READING

Hobbs CJ, Osman T. Genital injuries in boys and abuse. *Arch Dis Child* 2007;92(4):328–331.
Levey HR, Segal RL, Bivalacqua TJ. Management of priapism: An update for clinicians. *Ther Adv Urol* 2014;6(8):230–244.

PRECOCIOUS PUBERTY

Clinical Overview

Normal sexual development begins in girls with breast development, followed by the appearance of pubic hair (sometimes simultaneously with breast development), axillary hair, onset of menstruation, acne and adult body odour. In boys, it begins with testicular enlargement followed by enlargement of the penis, the appearance of pubic hair, deepening of the voice, acne and adult body odour. Precocious puberty (PP) is defined as puberty occurring at an unusual age, i.e. before the age of 8 years in girls or before 9 years in boys. Puberty nowadays starts earlier than in previous generations. Puberty depends on increased production of kisspeptin in the hypothalamus, resulting in increased gonadotropin-releasing hormone (GnRH), which acts on the pituitary gland to release gonadotropins luteinising hormone (LH) and follicle-stimulating hormone (FSH), which stimulate sex hormone production by the gonads. The causes of PP are best divided into gonadotropin-dependent central (idiopathic or with identifiable causes), gonadotropin-independent (adrenal and gonadal causes), or partial PP (thelarche, adrenarche, menarche). In more than 90% of girls and 50% of boys, the cause of PP is idiopathic, i.e. no identifiable cause. The main differentiating feature between central (hypothalamic) and adrenal causes is that the PP is always isosexual in the former and testes remain small in the latter cause.

Possible Diagnoses

Infants	Children
Common	
Central nervous system injury	Partial (incomplete) precocious puberty (PPP)
Adrenal (e.g. congenital adrenal)	Central idiopathic precocious puberty
Ovarian (e.g. McCune–Albright)	Central with identifiable causes (e.g. hypothalamic hamartoma)
Iatrogenic (external sex hormones)	Gonads (ovarian cysts, McCune–Albright syndrome)
PPP (e.g. premature thelarche)	Adrenal (e.g. congenital adrenal hyperplasia, tumour)
Rare	
	Iatrogenic (external sources of sex hormones)
	Irradiation of the brain
	Familial PP in males
	Teratoma (e.g. in the mediastinum)

Differential Diagnosis at a Glance

	PPP	Idiopathic Central PP	Central PP with a Cause	Gonad-Causing PP	Adrenal Causing PP
Normal growth	Yes	No	No	No	No
Gonadotropin dependent	No	Yes	Yes	No	No
More in girls than in boys	Yes	Yes	No	No	No
Advanced bone age	No	Yes	Yes	Yes	Yes
High FSH + LH	No	Yes	Yes	No	No

Recommended Investigations

*** Hormonal assay of GnRH, LH, FSH
*** GnRH stimulation test (in central PP, the LH and FSH levels are increased)
*** Serum level of I7-hydroxyprogesterone, dehydroepiandrosterone, cortisol and aldoste-
       rone in cases of CAH
*** Wrist X-ray to assess bone maturation
*** Pelvic ultrasound scan and adrenal visualisation for CAH
*** Cranial magnetic resonance imaging (MRI) for cases of suspected central PP
** Skeletal survey for bony fibrous dysplasia for a child with PP and hyperpigmented spots

Top Tips

- Puberty can easily be assessed by bone age: if bone age is within 1 year of chronological age, puberty either has not started or has just started; bone age within 2 years indicates the child is in puberty.
- Isolated thelarche is characterised by normal growth, age-appropriate skeletal maturation, pre-pubertal uterus and ovaries and isolated FSH elevation with pre-pubertal LH level.
- PPP is either an isolated breast development (precocious thelarche) or sexual hair appearance (precocious adrenarche) without other signs of puberty occurring before the age of 8 years in girls and 9 years in boys. PPP is usually benign and non-progressive. Onset younger than 3 years is frequently associated with regression over 1–3 years; later onset usually progresses slowly as PP.
- In precocious thelarche, the nipple is characteristically pale, immature, thin and transparent. In PP the nipple is mature and prominent with a dark areola indicating high circulating oestrogen.
- PP may have adverse effects on social behaviour and psychological development. An early growth spurt causes rapid bone maturation, resulting in early epiphyseal fusion and short stature.
- Low-dose radiation of the brain may induce PP in girls; high-dose radiation may induce PP in both sexes.
- Hypothyroidism can cause PP; children are, however, short and the growth velocity is decreased.
- Growth acceleration and advanced bone age (wrist X-ray) favour true PP against PPP.

Red Flags

- In any child with PP, careful search of the skin is essential: café-au-lait maculae with smooth borders suggest NF-1; larger café-au-lait patches with irregular outlines are consistent with McCune–Albright syndrome (polyostotic fibrous dysplasia of bone and ovarian cysts).
- Be aware that children with hypothalamic lesion may present with diabetes insipidus (polydipsia, polyuria), hyperthermia, obesity or loss of weight, or inappropriate crying or laughter.
- PP may put girls at risk of sexual abuse and psychological trauma from teasing and bullying.

- A child with precocious thelarche or adrenarche still needs careful evaluation, as these cannot often be easily and definitively differentiated from true PP.
- Full investigation, including imaging of the central nervous system and abdomen, should be carried out for all children with PP who have progressive signs of puberty, are younger than 8 years, with neurological signs or if the diagnosis is uncertain.
- Hypothalamic hamartoma (ectopic tissue secreting pulse GnRH) is the most common identifiable lesion causing PP. Examination of visual acuity, visual fields and eye fundi is essential.

FURTHER READING

Bajpal A, Menon PSN. Contemporary issues in precocious puberty. *Indian Endocrinol Metabol* 2011;15(Suppl 3):S172–S179.

Stephen MD, Zage PE, Waguespack SG. Gonadotropin-dependent precocious puberty: Neoplastic causes. *Int J Pediatr Endocrinol* 2011;2011(1):184502.

RECTAL PROLAPSE

Clinical Overview

Rectal prolapse (RP) refers to a herniation of the rectal mucosa through the anus. When the protrusion includes the rectal wall, it is termed *procidentia*. The mucosal type is the most common and least serious form of RP in children. Most cases of RP occur during the first few years of life, with a peak age of 1.5–6 years; it is rare in older children. It is usually noted after defaecation and is reduced either spontaneously or by the child's finger or parents. It rarely becomes chronic; if it does, complications such as ulceration, bleeding and inflammation (proctitis) are likely consequences. Most causes of RP are due to raised intra-abdominal pressure during chronic constipation, diarrhoea or cough. One of the most important causes of RP is cystic fibrosis (CF), and RP may be the first manifestation of the disease.

Possible Diagnoses

Infants	Children
Common	
CF	Idiopathic
Chronic diarrhoea (coeliac, infectious enteritis)	CF
Malnutrition	Chronic constipation
Idiopathic	Chronic diarrhoea (e.g. ulcerative colitis)
Parasitic infection	Connective tissue disorders (e.g. Ehlers-Danlos syndrome)
Rare	
Connective tissue disorders (CTDs)	Intestinal parasites
Chronic cough	Malnutrition
Repair of imperforate anus	Chronic cough (e.g. pertussis)
Meningomyelocele	Hirschsprung's disease
	Repair of imperforate anus
	Meningomyelocele

Differential Diagnosis at a Glance

	Idiopathic	CF	Constipation	Diarrhoea	Connective Tissue
History of excessive straining	Possible	No	Yes	Yes	No
Underweight	No	Possible	No	Yes	Possible
Clear cause from history	No	Yes	Yes	Yes	Possible
Other organ involvement	No	Yes	Possible	Possible	Yes
Good disease outcome	Yes	No	Yes	Possible	No

Recommended Investigations

- *** Screening tests in blood for coeliac disease (CD)
- *** Stool for culture, search for parasites
- *** Chest X-ray and nasopharyngeal swab in cases with chronic cough
- *** Sweat test for CF
- *** Rectoscopy/sigmoidoscopy with possible biopsy for cases with chronic diarrhoea (e.g. ulcerative colitis)

Top Tips

- RP is more common in tropical and developing countries, due to high prevalence of diarrhoea, malnutrition and parasitic infestation.
- Prolonged sitting on a child's potty and straining predisposes for RP; these should be avoided.
- Once the cause of the RP is established, the best advice is not to panic; the RP is likely to recur.
- Parents and affected older children have to be taught how to reduce prolapse at home and told to seek medical assistance if this is not achieved.
- Solitary rectal ulcer syndrome manifests as rectal bleeding, constipation, prolonged straining, mucous discharge and PR. The condition should not be misdiagnosed as inflammatory bowel disease, polyps or complication from PR.
- Remember that CF is one of the most common causes of RP; about 20% of CF patients have RP.
- In contrast to adults, incidence and recurrence of RP decrease as children grow older, and conservative management is usually successful and indicated.

Red Flags

- RP is usually painless or associated with mild discomfort; pain suggests complications such as ulceration, ischaemia or proctitis.
- A sweat test is indicated in all children with RP who present without a known underlying cause.
- RP has to be differentiated from rarer causes of prolapse resembling RP: prolapsed intussusception, haemorrhoids and prolapsed polyp. The latter appears as a dark, plum-coloured mass in contrast to the lighter pink mucosa appearance of the RP.
- Prolonged straining at defecation is a major cause for RP.
- Some mothers insist on placing the child, even an infant, on a potty to strain for a long period. This puts the child at risk for RP.

FURTHER READING

Urganci N, Kalyon CV, Ekes KG. Solitary rectal ulcer syndrome in children: A report of six cases. *Gut Liver* 2013;7(6):752–755.

SCROTAL/TESTICULAR SWELLING

Clinical Overview

Following completion of testicular descent, the processus vaginalis closes and its lower portion becomes the tunica vaginalis testis. Failure to close results in a patent processus allowing the development of the two most common causes of painless scrotal swelling: hydrocele and inguinal hernia. Hydrocele is caused by drainage of peritoneal fluid through a narrow patent processus vaginalis (communicating hydrocele), while a wide patent processus vaginalis causes inguinal hernia by allowing omentum or bowel to pass into the scrotum. Failure to close the processus vaginalis in females results in formation of a patent pouch of the peritoneum with possible complication of inguinal hernia and hydrocele (hydrocele of canal of Nuck). The four most common painful causes of testicular swelling are testicular torsion, torsion of testicular appendage, incarcerated inguinal hernia and epididymitis/orchitis. Children with any of these causes may present as an acute scrotum, which is a medical emergency defined as scrotal pain, swelling and redness.

Possible Diagnoses

Infants	Children
Common	
Hydrocele	Hydrocele
Inguinal hernia	Inguinal hernia
Birth trauma affecting the genitalia	Testicular torsion
Epididymitis/orchitis	Epididymitis/orchitis
Drainage from ascites	Hydrocele of spermatic cord
Rare	
Testicular torsion	Testicular tumour (germ tumour)
Generalised oedema (e.g. nephrotic syndrome)	Trauma (scrotal haematoma)
Testicular tumour (e.g. hamartoma)	Idiopathic scrotal oedema (ISO)
	Generalised oedema
	Torsion of the spermatic cord
	Varicocele
	Vasculitis (HSP)

Differential Diagnosis at a Glance

	Hydrocele	Inguinal Hernia	Testicular Torsion	Orchitis/ Epididymitis	Hydrocele Spermatic Cord
Acute onset	No	No	Yes	Yes	No
Pain/tender	No	No	Yes	Yes	No
Ill looking	No	No	Yes	Yes	No
Fever/vomit	No	No	Yes	Possible	No
Trans-illumination	Yes	Yes	No	No	Yes

Recommended Investigations

*** Urinalysis may suggest associated urinary tract infection (UTI) in epididymitis, proteinuria for NS

*** Plasma albumin, urea and electrolytes and cholesterol for NS

** Plasma α-fetoprotein for any malignant testicular tumour (usually elevated)
** Ultrasonography helps whether testis is present or merely hydrocele
** Colour Doppler ultrasonography assesses the testicular morphology and testicular blood flow
** CT or MRI may delineate some testicular tumour pre-operatively

Top Tips

- Virtually all hydroceles are congenital in neonates and infants. In a mobile child with hydrocele, the size characteristically increases during daytime and decreases over nighttime.
- Spermatic cord hydrocele is uncommon and results from aberration in the closure of the processus vaginalis. It is a loculated fluid collection along the spermatic cord, separated from the testis and epididymis and located above them.
- Torsion of testicular appendix can be differentiated from testicular torsion by the blue dot sign, which is a necrotic appendage after undergoing torsion.
- Epididymitis is the most common cause of scrotal swelling in sexually active young adolescents. This is an ascending infection from the urethra.
- ISO, usually caused by allergy, may mimic torsion. The scrotum is swollen and red in ISO, there are no symptoms, and the testis characteristically feels normal and not tender. ISO often extends to the groin and perineum. Parents can be reassured that the swelling will disappear within a few days (without treatment), leaving some purpuric discolouration.
- Varicocele occurs in about 5% of all adolescent boys and is a common cause of subfertility.

Red Flags

- In the normal scrotum, 1–2 mL of serous fluid is present in the tunica vaginalis and should not be mistaken for hydrocele.
- Acquired hydrocele can decrease the efficiency of spermatogenesis by causing atrophic changes due to increased pressure on the blood supply of the testis. In addition, tumours of the tunica vaginalis may be obscured by hydrocele, hence the need for rapid treatment.
- It is critical to determine whether a scrotal mass is intra- or extra-testicular. The majority of intra-testicular masses are malignant, while extra-testicular masses are usually benign.
- Be aware that torsion of testis in neonates may be asymptomatic except for red scrotal swelling.
- In a suspected case of testicular torsion, clinicians should not request any imaging or test. The diagnosis is clinical and imaging is unnecessary. Surgical exploration is urgent.
- Abrupt onset of painful scrotal swelling is usually caused by incarcerated hernia or testicular torsion. The onset of pain in torsion of testicular appendix is usually gradual.
- Epididymitis/orchitis may mimic testicular torsion; the inflammation, however, is commonly secondary to viral infection (e.g. mumps) or sexually transmitted disease (STD). In addition, the pain is more gradual in epididymitis/orchitis and nausea and vomiting is uncommon, often with fever, dysuria and pyuria.

FURTHER READING

Dagur G, Gandhi J, Suh Y et al. Classifying hydroceles of the pelvis and groin: An overview of the etiology, secondary complications, evaluation and management. *Curr Urol* 2017;10(1):1–14.

VAGINAL DISCHARGE

Clinical Overview

Vaginal discharge (VD) is the most common gynaecological problem in pre-pubertal children and adolescents. Physiologically, it occurs in neonate girls who often experience vaginal discharge (pseudo-menstruation) as a result of withdrawal of the maternal oestrogen hormone. A rise of oestrogen at the onset of puberty causes another physiological discharge (leucorrhoea). Pathological conditions of VD include non-specific VD (occurring in up to 70% of girls), which is caused by poor perineal hygiene, tendency of the labia minora to open on squatting, and close proximity of the anal orifice to the vagina allowing transfer of faecal bacteria to the vagina. Other contributory factors include the use of systemic antibiotics and steroids, wearing tight-fitting clothes such as tights, and the use of irritants such as detergents and bubble bath. Children with VD present with pruritus, frequent urination, dysuria, enuresis, sleep disturbance or erythema of the vulva. Sexual abuse is a serious problem and a high index of suspicion is required to make the diagnosis.

Possible Diagnoses

Infants	Children
Common	
Physiological	Physiological VD
Candida infection	Non-specific vulvovaginitis
Seborrhoeic dermatitis	STD
Atopic dermatitis	Foreign body (FB)
Vulvar psoriasis	Child abuse
Rare	
Urethral prolapse	*Candida* infection
Threadworms	Contact and allergic dermatitis
	Threadworms
	Lichen sclerosus
	Lichen planus
	Scabies
	Urethral prolapse
	Rhabdomyosarcoma

Differential Diagnosis at a Glance

	Physiological	Vulvovaginitis	STD	Foreign Body	Sexual Abuse
Foul odour	No	Possible	Yes	Yes	Possible
Associated erythema	No	Yes	Yes	Possible	Possible
Positive bacteria finding	No	Possible	Yes	Possible	Possible
Tear laceration	No	No	Possible	Possible	Yes
Adolescent age	Possible	No	Yes	Possible	No

Recommended Investigations

*** Urine sample for dipsticks and urine culture for suspected UTI
*** Swab from the discharge for Gram stain and culture, and for *Candida*

** Adhesive tape test to detect worm ova
** Imaging occasionally is required, e.g. for suspected FB or tumour

Top Tips

- The non-specific discharge of VD is typically brown or green and has a mild foetid odour. It may be associated with bacterial infection secondary to faecal contamination.
- Threadworm infection typically causes recurrent vulvovaginitis and manifests as nocturnal scratching due to female worms depositing eggs on the perineum.
- Discharge caused by *Candida* infection is rare before puberty but may occur in infancy. Risk factors in later age include systemic use of antibiotics and steroids.
- Child abuse refers to the use of children in sexual activities (including fondling, masturbation, penetration) that they do not understand or give consent to.
- Note that the majority of cases of physical examination on children suspected of child abuse do not yield abnormal findings. This does not exclude child abuse.
- Lichen sclerosus is characterised by a sharply demarcated area of hypopigmentation around the vulva and the perianal area. It is associated with intense itching and bleeds easily with normal toilet activities such as genital wiping.

Red Flags

- The physiological discharge and bleeding in neonate girls is usually creamy white and subsides when the child is 2 weeks old. Any discharge or bleeding after 2–3 weeks warrants investigation.
- FB should be considered when the discharge has a foul odour. Common objects include clumped toilet tissue or small parts of toys. Examination under general anaesthesia may be indicated.
- Children suffering from child abuse may present with symptoms not related directly to their genitalia, e.g. sleep disturbance, behaviour changes, phobias, anorexia, poor school performance and social withdrawal. Later on, victims often present with post-traumatic stress disorder.
- The interview of the child suspected of being sexually abused is the most valuable component of medical evaluation, using the child's words for body parts, drawings and age-appropriate questions. Clinicians should not conduct the interview unless they have skill and experience.
- Beware that most perpetrators of child abuse are family members, close relatives or friends who typically began relating to the child during non-sexual activities to gain the child's trust.
- UTI and threadworm infection are common in cases of VD. Unless the UTI and threadworms are treated, treatment for VD is inadequate and VD will recur.

FURTHER READING

Ganguli S, Liu Q, Tsoumpariotis A et al. Vaginal discharge in a prepubertal girl posing a diagnostic challenge. *Cureus* 2018;10(4):e2424.
Stricker T, Navratil F, Sennhauser FH. Vulvovaginitis in prepubertal girls. *Arch Dis Child* 2003;88:324–326.

12 CEREBRAL

ACUTE CONFUSIONAL STATE

Clinical Overview

Acute confusional state (ACS) is characterised by sudden alteration of the mental state leading to an inappropriate interaction with people and environment. It is characterised by an acute and dramatic onset of disorientation, impaired concentration and subtle motor signs such as tremor. Disorientation in older children is most marked for time. A child presenting with ACS should be regarded as a medical emergency. In the absence of a relevant medical history (such as sickle-cell anaemia or medication), the differential diagnosis can be quite difficult and challenging for clinicians to make. Although delirium is sometimes called ACS, in delirium, there is extreme disturbance of arousal, attention, orientation and perception, commonly accompanied by fear and agitation. Delirium is often associated with high fever which accompanies viral or bacterial infection, e.g. pneumonia. In infants, ACS occurs as an alteration of consciousness and is discussed later in this section.

Possible Diagnoses

Infants	Children
Common	
See sections on "Coma" and "Transient Loss of Consciousness"	Migraine
	Side effect of medication (e.g. antihistamine)
	Encephalitis/encephalopathy
	Non-convulsive status epilepticus (NCSE)
	Psychosis
	Concussion
	Drug ingestion
Rare	
	High fever
	Traumatic brain injury
	Hypoglycaemia
	Brain tumour, haemorrhage
	Night terror
	Systemic lupus erythematosus (SLE)
	Metabolic disorder (e.g. urea cycle disorder)
	Malignant hypertension
	Cerebral venous sinus thrombosis
	Carbon monoxide poisoning

Differential Diagnosis at a Glance

	Migraine	Medication	Encephalitis	NCSE	Psychosis
Positive family history	Yes	No	No	Possible	Possible
Previous/current hallucination, delusion	No	No	No	No	Yes
Subtle movements	No	Possible	Possible	Yes	Possible
Associated headache	Yes	No	Possible	No	Possible
Abnormal electroencephalogram (EEG)	No	No	Yes	Yes	No

Recommended Investigations

*** Blood glucose to exclude hypoglycaemia
*** Serological tests to exclude SLE
*** EEG for seizure (such as NCSE) or encephalitis
*** Neuroimaging with magnetic resonance imaging (MRI) or computed tomography (CT) scan for head injury, encephalitis (herpetic encephalitis)

Top Tips

• Nearly 10% of patients with migraine may present with migraine variants of which 5% develop ACS. Typically patients present with agitation, disorientation, speech difficulties and memory loss. The majority complained of headache prior to the confusion.
• EEG is diagnostic in NCSE: IV anti-epileptic drugs will normalise the EEG and resolve the ACS.
• The first step in evaluating any child with psychosis is to ask: is the child on any medication? In adolescence, illicit drugs (cocaine, amphetamine and ecstasy) are a common cause.
• Psychosis has numerous neurological causes including brain tumour, central nervous system infection and, most important in adolescents, drugs such as amphetamine, cocaine and ecstasy. Mental psychosis should include symptoms such as delusion, hallucination and paranoid ideation.
• Haloperidol is often used to treat ACS. The drug can cause unpleasant extra-pyramidal side effects. Procyclidine is an effective antidote.

Red Flags

• A confusional state of migraine often lasts several minutes to hours. It may be the first presentation before the onset of typical migraine attacks.
• The diagnosis of the first episode of acute confusional migraine is often difficult, particularly if a patient presents with symptoms such as sudden blindness, numbness or paraesthesias.
• Be aware that minor trauma can occasionally trigger a major ACS grossly disproportionate to the degree of trauma.
• NCSE should be considered in all children with ACS even if there is no history of epilepsy.
• Beware that patients with SLE may present initially with psychotic manifestations (personality changes, depression and agitation) before occurrence of classical features (e.g. malar rash).

FURTHER READING

Faroogi AM, Padilla JM, Monteith TS. Acute confusional migraine: Distinct clinical or spectrum of migraine biology? *Brain Sci* 2018;8(2):29.

DEVELOPMENTAL DISABILITY

Clinical Overview

Developmental disability (DD) is a heterogeneous group of chronic conditions that include problems in cognitive functioning, physical functioning or both. Intellectual disability (or intellectual developmental disorder) encompasses the cognitive part, which is broadly related to thought process. DD results in limitation in areas of normal activities, including communication, self-care, social adaptation and physical functioning. The condition is common affecting about 3% of the population, of which over 90% are categorised as mild and about 5% as severe or profound. Most children with mild disability are identified in the pre-school period because of the inability to communicate, inability to take care of oneself (including decision-making) and deficiency in participating in social and school activities. Traditionally, DD has been grouped as prenatal (e.g. chromosomal, genetic disorder, toxins or infection during pregnancy), natal (e.g. prematurity, hypoxic-ischaemic encephalopathy [HIE], infection) and postnatal causes (e.g. head injury, autism and infection).

Possible Diagnoses

Infants	Children
Common	
Extreme prematurity	Chromosomal (trisomy-21, fragile X syndrome)
Intracranial haemorrhage	Idiopathic (cause unidentified)
Infection (e.g. toxoplasmosis, rubella, cytomegalovirus and herpes [TORCH], meningitis)	Cerebral palsy (CP)
Metabolic (e.g. hypoglycaemia)	Autism spectrum disorder
HIE	Traumatic brain injury
Rare	
Inborn errors of metabolism	Genetic syndrome (e.g. fragile X syndrome)
Primary microcephaly	Post-infection
Congenital central nervous system (CNS) malformation	Neurocutaneous syndrome (e.g. tuberous sclerosis)
Seizures (e.g. infantile spasm)	Child abuse
Fetal alcohol syndrome	Metabolic (hypoglycaemia, hypernatraemia)
Child abuse (physical, neglect)	Toxins (e.g. lead)
	Mucopolysaccharidosis, galactosaemia
	Inborn errors of metabolism
	Long-term malnutrition

Differential Diagnosis at a Glance

	Chromosomal	Idiopathic	CP	Autism	Head Injury
Identified at birth	Yes	Possible	No	No	No
Severe DD	Yes	Possible	Possible	Possible	Possible
Acute onset	No	No	Possible	No	Yes
Motor disability	Possible	Possible	Possible	No	Possible
Associated ID	Yes	Possible	Possible	Yes	Possible

Recommended Investigations

***   Urine for mucopolysaccharides; reducing substance for galactosaemia
***   Metabolic screen: blood glucose, urea and electrolytes, organic acids, amino acids, ammonia
**   Serum uric acid for any boy with self-mutilation (Lesch-Nyhan syndrome)
**   Blood lead, serum copper and ceruloplasmin for Wilson's disease
**   Serological and microbiological studies for congenital (TORCH) infection
**   White blood cell lysosomal enzyme or skin biopsy for neuro-regression, optic atrophy
***   Genetic studies (e.g. microarray, gene panel, exome or genome sequencing) for DD, ID, autism spectrum disorder or congenital anomalies
***   EEG for associated seizure disorders
***   Cranial MRI for focal seizures, neurocutaneous syndrome

Top Tips

- Mild degree of DD may not manifest until toddler age or after school entry and is usually present with delayed speech and language development.
- The long-used classification of DD based on IQ (mild: 55–69; moderate: 40–54; severe: <40) is no longer used. New classification of DD was based on the amount of support and supervision that the individual needs: intermittent, limited, extensive and pervasive.
- The term *mental retardation* should not be used because of undesirable stigma. Intellectual disability, developmental delay or learning difficulty are more appropriate terms.
- CP is the most common cause of physical disability characterised by significant impairment in movement and posture that begins in infancy or early childhood.
- Chromosomal microarray (CMA) should be the first test in the genetic evaluation of children with DD including ID and autism spectrum disorder.
- Neglect (e.g. isolation, bullying) or child abuse is recognised to cause DD. Neglect is three times more common than physical abuse and tends to occur over a long period of time.

Red Flags

- In a child with suspected DD: is the hearing and vision normal? Inability to identify visual or hearing impairment causes social isolation and psychological and emotional problems.
- Be aware of the difference between a child who has always had developmental disability and one who developed normally and then lost motor or cognitive skill. The latter needs an urgent evaluation as such regression may indicate a neurodegenerative disease.
- Red flags in suspected CP include a child not sitting by 8 months, not walking by 18 months, the presence of severe symptoms in the absence of a history of perinatal injury, muscular hypotonia, paraplegia, normal MRI and abnormal basal ganglia imaging.
- Remember that toe walking is normal for several months in toddlers. Any persistent toe walking requires referral.
- Fragile X syndrome is seen in 1 in 2,600 males and 1 in 4,200 females. Affected children exhibit delayed speech and poor eye contact that are often wrongly mistaken as signs of autism.

FURTHER READING

Lee RW, Poretti A, Cohen JS et al. A diagnostic approach for cerebral palsy in the genomic era. *Neuromuscular Med* 2014;18(4):821–844.

Maenner MJ, Blumberg SJ, Kogan MD et al. Prevalence of cerebral palsy and intellectual disability among children identified in two US national surveys. *Ann Epidemiol* 2016;26(3):2011–2013.

National Institute for Health and Care Excellence (NICE). Cerebral palsy in under 25s: Assessment and management. *NICE guideline 2017 (NG62)*. https://www.nice.org.uk/guidance/ng62

HEADACHE

Clinical Overview

Headache is a common symptom in children, occurring in about 50% of children aged 7 years and 80% of children aged 15 years. It may be acute, acute recurrent, chronic recurrent or progressive, caused by minor viral infections or severe underlying disease such as CNS infection or increased intracranial pressure (ICP). Therefore, careful evaluation of a child with headache is essential. Infants or toddlers with headache present with irritability, unwillingness to play, crying while holding the head or vomiting. The most common causes of headache are acute viral infection, migraine and tension headache. Migraine without aura is the most common type, defined as a headache lasting 1–72 hours, plus two of the following: bilateral or unilateral, pulsating, aggravated by routine physical activities, plus at least one of the following: nausea and/or vomiting, photophobia or phonophobia. Tension headache is diagnosed as headache lasting from 30 minutes to 7 days, in addition to two of the following: pressing/tightening, non-pulsating, mild–moderate intensity, bilateral with no nausea or vomiting.

Possible Diagnoses

Infants	Children
Common	
Birth trauma causing cerebral irritability	Common viral infections
Viral infection	Migraine
Migraine	Tension headache
Head injury	Brain lesions (e.g. tumour, haemorrhage)
Subdural haematoma (e.g. child abuse)	Sinusitis
	Medication overuse
Rare	
CNS infection	Eye strain
Increased ICP	CNS infection (meningitis, brain abscess)
	Mitochondrial disease such as mitochondrial encephalopathy, lactic acidosis and stroke-like episodes (MELAS)
	Traumatic brain injury
	Medications
	Seizure
	Hypertension
	Benign increased ICP (pseudotumour cerebri)

Differential Diagnosis at a Glance

	Viral Infection	Migraine	Tension Headache	Brain Lesion	Sinusitis
Normal daily activities	Yes	No	Possible	No	Possible
Associated fever	Possible	No	No	No	Yes
Lasts less than 1 hour	Yes	No	Possible	No	Possible
Morning symptoms	No	No	Possible	Yes	Possible
Recurring	No	Yes	Yes	No	No

Recommended Investigations

The vast majority of children presenting with headaches do not require any investigation. The indication to use neuroimaging is discussed in this section.

Top Tips

- It is simple to differentiate the two most common causes of headaches: migraine disrupts the child's activity; tension headache does not.
- In families with a history of migraine, migraine variants are common and include cyclic vomiting, paroxysmal vertigo, restless legs, paroxysmal torticollis and abdominal migraine.
- Recurrent headache such as migraine is more than just a painful episode; it is often accompanied by impaired academic performance, school absences, disturbed sleep and poor quality of life.
- In contrast to adults with migraine, childhood migraine tends to be shorter in duration (1–48 hours), often bilateral (frontal or bitemporal) with gastrointestinal symptoms, e.g. abdominal pain.
- Although analgesics such as paracetamol, ibuprofen and sumatriptan are effective first-line treatments in migraine, evidence-based treatment or prophylaxis is lacking. Prophylaxis is considered for missing more than 3 days of school in a month and/or one to two attacks per week.
- A history of analgesic overuse can be a contributory factor in headache chronicity because the headache may be analgesic induced. Discontinuation of the analgesics improves the headache.
- Benign increased ICP (pseudotumour cerebri) is characterised by increased ICP (e.g. headaches, vomiting and papilloedema) with normal CSF and ventricular size. Focal neurological signs are absent.

Red Flags

- Symptoms that require urgent attention include headaches that wake a child from sleep, early morning vomiting without nausea, worsening headache, associated personality changes or neurological symptoms.
- Be aware that frequent headache, including migraine, may be caused by emotional, sexual and physical child abuse.
- Basilar migraine (presenting with vertigo, diplopia, blurred vision, ataxia) should be differentiated from posterior fossa tumour.
- Headache in association with other neurological symptoms is common in brain tumours, but headache may be the only symptom in some brain tumours.
- In an infant with cerebral haematoma, child abuse should be considered. Children may present with irritability, vomiting, bulging fontanelle and focal seizure. Fundoscopy may show retinal haemorrhage. Neuroimaging is urgent.
- Remember that MELAS may present with recurrent migraine-like headaches.

FURTHER READING

Shankin CJ, Ferrari U, Reinisch VM et al. Characteristics of brain tumour-associated headache. *Cephalalgia* 2007;27(7):204–911.
Tietjen GE, Buse DC, Fanning KM et al. Recalled maltreatment, migraine, and tension-type headache. *Neurology* 2015;84(2):132–140.

FAINTING (TRANSIENT LOSS OF CONSCIOUSNESS)

Clinical Overview

Normally, standing is associated with a transfer of blood to the legs causing transient instability and a drop of blood pressure (BP) for 10–20 seconds. Reflex tachycardia and vasoconstriction restore BP within 30–60 seconds. Transient loss of consciousness, often referred to as blackout, is common in children and includes syncope, epileptic causes and non-epileptic causes. Syncope is by far the most common cause with a lifetime incidence of about 40%. It is defined as transient and self-limited loss of consciousness and postural tone due to transient cerebral hypoperfusion. It is characterised by rapid onset, short duration and spontaneous complete recovery. Orthostatic hypotension denotes fall of BP on standing. Neurogenic orthostatic hypotension is due to impaired sympathetic activation with a fall in BP with little or no increase in heart rate (HR). In non-neurogenic orthostatic hypotension, sympathetic activation is normal, leading to tachycardia and hypotension. Postural tachycardia syndrome (POTS), common in persons with migraine, is characterised by excessive increase in HR after a few minutes' standing while BP is minimally changed. As a significant number of patients with syncope are misdiagnosed with epilepsy with serious implications on the patients' life, epilepsy is included in this section.

Possible Diagnoses

Infants	Children
Common	
Cardiac arrhythmia	Syncope (vasovagal faint)
	Seizure (epilepsy)
	Cardiac syncope
	Orthostatic hypotension (neurogenic and non-neurogenic)
	POTS
Rare	
	Toxins/poisoning/medication
	Pulmonary hypertension
	Mastocytosis
	Takayasu arteritis (large vessel vasculitis)
	Cardiac arrhythmia (e.g. long QT syndrome)

Differential Diagnosis at a Glance

	Syncope	Seizure	Cardiac Syncope	Orthostatic Hypotension	POTS
Occurs mainly in upright position	Yes	No	No	Yes	Yes
Abnormal high pulse on standing	Possible	No	No	Possible	Yes
Commonly older than 10 years	Yes	No	No	Yes	Yes
Low BP on immediate standing	Yes	No	No	Possible	No
Diagnosis by electrocardiogram (ECG) or EEG	No	Yes	Yes	No	Possible

Recommended Investigations

*** Full blood count (FBC) and C-reactive protein (CRP): leukocytosis and high CRP in infection
*** Lumbar puncture and blood culture (BC) for CNS infection
*** Blood sugar (BS) (Boehringer Mannheim (producing blood glucose test strips) [BM] stick) to diagnose hyper- or hypoglycaemia
*** Tilt-table testing: very useful in children with unexplained syncope
*** ECG in fainting to exclude long QT syndrome; event monitor or 24 hour ECG may be necessary
*** Plain X-ray for skull injury, skeletal survey for suspected abuse
*** EEG and neuroimaging for suspected epilepsy, haemorrhage or mass

Top Tips

- Most causes of impaired consciousness can be diagnosed from the history alone; an eye-witness account is essential, e.g. if the event occurred at school, a report from there is required.
- Examination of a child with fainting includes supine value of HR and BP at 1 and 3 minutes, followed by standing measurement of HR and BP at 1 and 3 minutes. A HR of >30 beats/min between supine and standing suggests POTS.
- ECG is an essential tool to examine children with syncope, possibly diagnosing WPW (Wolff–Parkinson–White) syndrome, long QT syndrome, T-wave inversion, and ventricular hypertrophy.

Red Flags

- Vasovagal syncope may be associated with brief limb twitching, upward eye deviation, and even urinary incontinence. These should not be misdiagnosed as epilepsy. Failure to recognise these features often leads to wrong diagnosis and unnecessary administration of anti-epileptic drugs.
- QTc duration >480 msec finding in the ECG is a significant predictor for first syncope and patients are at high risk for the development of subsequent syncope and fatal/near-fatal events.
- Arrhythmias are an important cause of loss of consciousness and possible death; urgent referral to a cardiologist is indicated for consideration of treatment with β-blockers. In refractory cases an implantable pacemaker may be considered.
- Sudden unexplained death in the young has devastating effects on surviving family members. Death may be due to long QT syndrome, hypertrophic cardiomyopathy or Brugada syndrome. Family screening is required.
- Before diagnosing epilepsy, consider conditions that mimic seizures such as breath-holding spells, syncope, narcolepsy and pseudo-seizure. Remember that the latter frequently occurs in patients with a past history of epilepsy. EEG and serum prolactin (increased in true epilepsy) help.

FURTHER READING

Colan S. Hypertrophic cardiomyopathy in children. *Heart Fail Clin* 2010;6(4):433–444.
Liu JF, Jons L, Moss AJ et al. Risk factors for recurrent syncope and subsequent fatal or near-fatal events in children and adolescents with long QT syndrome. *J Am Coll Cardiol* 2011;57(8):941–950.

COMA

Clinical Overview

Prolonged and deeper impaired consciousness (coma) usually results from traumatic brain injury, or intracranial (e.g. infection) or metabolic (e.g. diabetic ketoacidosis) disorders. Cerebral malaria and traumatic brain injury are the most common causes of coma worldwide. Traumatic head injury, defined as injury to the scalp, skull or brain, is a common event, and brain injuries are the most frequent cause of trauma fatality among children. Compared to adults, children have higher brain water content, the size of the head is relatively larger than the rest of the body, and vasculature is easily disrupted, hence the higher risk of epidural and subdural haematoma.

Possible Diagnoses

Infants	Children
Common	
Hypoxic-ischaemic encephalopathy	Traumatic brain injury
Seizures	Seizure (epilepsy)
Traumatic brain injury	Cerebral malaria
Urea cycle disorder	Infection (encephalitis)
Intracranial infection	Drug toxicity
Rare	
Toxins/poisoning/medication	Diabetic ketoacidosis (DKA)/hypoglycaemia
Sudden infant death syndrome	Hysteria
	Reye's syndrome
	Intracranial haemorrhage (e.g. stroke)
	Electrolytes disturbance (e.g. hyponatraemia)
	Cardiac arrhythmia

Differential Diagnosis at a Glance

	Head Injury	Seizure	Cerebral Malaria	Infection	Drug Toxicity
History of trauma	Yes	No	No	No	No
In tropics	Possible	Possible	Yes	Yes	Possible
Previous similar event	No	Possible	No	No	Possible
Presence of fever	No	No	Yes	Yes	Possible
Diagnosis by EEG	No	Yes	No	No	No

Recommended Investigations

- *** FBC and CRP: leukocytosis and high CRP in infection
- *** Lumbar puncture and BC for CNS infection
- *** BS (BM stick) to diagnose hyper- or hypoglycaemia
- *** Tilt-table testing: very useful in children with unexplained syncope
- *** ECG in fainting to exclude prolonged QT; 24-hour continuous ECG is often required
- *** Plain X-ray for skull injury, skeletal survey for suspected abuse
- *** EEG and neuroimaging for suspected epilepsy, haemorrhage or mass

Top Tips

- Most causes of impaired consciousness can be diagnosed from the history alone; so an eyewitness account is essential.
- The Glasgow coma scale is a valuable tool in assessing children with an altered level of consciousness, particularly in cases with head trauma.
- Ornithine transcarbamylase deficiency (OTCD) is the most common urea cycle disorder presenting during the neonatal period with an acute hyper-ammonaemic coma, with lethargy, failure to thrive and vomiting.
- The main strategy of management for mild head injury is rest and observation for 24–48 hours.
- Hyperglycaemia hyperosmolar state (HHS) is defined as serum glucose >600 mg/dL, serum osmolality >330 mOsm/kg, without significant ketosis or acidosis.

Red Flags

- In children with head injury: life-threatening injury includes Glasgow coma scale <15, 2 hours after injury, open or depressed skull fracture, worsening headache and irritability, basal skull fracture.
- Be suspicious of head injury in infants: the majority of serious intracranial injuries (excluding road traffic accidents) during the first year of life are due to abuse.
- Before diagnosing epilepsy, consider conditions that mimic seizures such as breath-holding spells, syncope, narcolepsy and pseudo-seizure. Remember that the latter frequently occurs in patients with a past history of epilepsy. EEG and serum prolactin (increased in true epilepsy) help.
- In any well neonate at birth who then becomes lethargic and vomits, OTCD must be excluded. Immediate serum ammonia level measurement and dietary protein withdrawal are essential.
- Seizures are common in comatose children; they can be extremely subtle and only diagnosed by EEG.
- Although DKA and HHS may overlap, DKA must be differentiated from HHS because patients with HHS are severely dehydrated and require more aggressive fluid therapy.

FURTHER READING

Chiang JL, Kirkman MS, Laffel LMB et al. Type 1 diabetes through the life span: A position statement of the American Diabetes Association. *Diabetes Care* 2014;37(7):2034–2054.

Garcia-Rodriguez JA, Thomas RE. Office management of mild head injury in children and adolescents. *Can Fam Physician* 2014;60(6):523–531.

Garg K, Sharma R, Gupta D et al. Outcome predictors in pediatric head trauma: A study of clinico-radiological factors. *J Pediatr Neurosci* 2017;12(2):149–153.

NEUROMUSCULAR WEAKNESS

Clinical Overview

Acquired and hereditary neuromuscular diseases are characterised by an abnormality of any component of the lower motor neurone (LMN): anterior horn cell (e.g. spinal muscular atrophy), peripheral nerve (e.g. Guillain–Barré syndrome [GBS]), neuromuscular junction (e.g. myasthenia gravis) and muscle including muscular dystrophies (e.g. Duchenne muscular dystrophy [DMD]) and myopathies (congenital myotonia, mitochondrial disease). LMN lesion may manifest as normal intellect, markedly reduced muscle power (paralysis), reduced muscle bulk and reduced muscle tone often with diminished reflexes and presence of fasciculation (present with anterior horn cell disease). Diseases of the LMN may be inherited or acquired, with acute onset within days or weeks (poliomyelitis, GBS) or chronic. Weakness must be differentiated from hypotonia, fatigue and ataxia.

Possible Diagnoses

Infants	Children
Common	
Spinal muscular atrophy	Spinal muscular atrophy (SMA)
	Peripheral nerve (e.g. Guillain–Barré syndrome)
Congenital myasthenia	Neuromuscular junction (e.g. myasthenia gravis)
Congenital muscular dystrophy	Muscular dystrophy (e.g. DMD)
Congenital myopathies	Congenital myopathy
Rare	
Familial dysautonomia (Riley-Day syndrome)	Dermatomyositis
Infant botulism	Metabolic myopathies
	Spinal tumour
	Botulism
	Acute flaccid myelitis
	Endocrine myopathy (e.g. hypothyroidism)
	Periodic paralysis (hyper- and hypokalaemic)
	Drugs (e.g. steroids)
	Motor neurone disease
	Transient myelitis

Differential Diagnosis at a Glance

	SMA	Guillain–Barré Syndrome	Myasthenia	DMD	Myopathy
Acute onset	No	Yes	No	No	Possible
Early facial involvement	No	No	Yes	No	Yes
Calf hypertrophy	No	No	No	Yes	No
Fasciculation	Yes	No	No	No	No
High serum creatinine kinase (CK)	No	No	No	Yes	No

Recommended Investigations

*** Serum electrolytes for unexplained episodic paralysis
*** Thyroid function test in suspected thyroid-related disorders

***   Serum creatinine phosphokinase for muscle diseases such as DMD
**   Serum lactate and pyruvate for mitochondrial disease
***   Anti-acetylcholine receptor or anti-muscle specific kinase antibody in serum or plasma
       and edrophonium or neostigmine test may confirm myasthenia gravis
***   ECG monitoring for cardiac involvement, e.g. DMD
***   EMG can differentiate between neuropathic and myopathic disorders
**   Muscle biopsy

Top Tips

- Examination of a child with weakness should always begin with observation, including the head (shape and size), face (for dysmorphism), eyes (for strabismus, ophthalmoplegia), skin, and muscles (for any lesion, atrophy, hypertrophy, fasciculation) and gait (waddling, ataxic), and whether there is difficulty in rising up from the floor.
- Remember that proximal muscle weakness (shoulders and hips) indicates a myopathy, while distal weakness (hands) indicates a neuropathy. Myotonic dystrophy is an exception, with weakness affecting the hands.
- Children with congenital myopathies are distinguished from muscular dystrophies by facial weakness and normal or mildly elevated serum CK level.
- Both hypothyroidism and hyperthyroidism can cause proximal muscle myopathies; patients with Grave's disease may cause ophthalmoplegia.

Red Flags

- Infant botulism should be considered in infants with acute bulbar dysfunction and hypotonia.
- In a boy with an inability to walk by the age of 18 months, DMD has to be excluded by serum CK.
- Children with periodic paralysis are normal between episodes. Later these become more frequent, causing permanent weakness.
- Children with leukodystrophies may cause diagnostic confusion as they have both upper and lower motor lesions.

FURTHER READING

Dowling JJ, Gonorazky HD, Cohn RD et al. Treating pediatric neuromuscular disorders: The future is now. *Am J Med Genet A* 2018;176(4):804–841.
McDonald CM. Clinical approach to the diagnostic evaluation of hereditary and acquired neuromuscular diseases. *Phys Med Rehabil Clin N Am* 2012;23(3):495–563.
Nayak R. Practical approach to the patient with acute neuromuscular weakness. *World J Clin Cases* 2017;5(7):270–279.

SEIZURE

Clinical Overview

The term *seizure* is preferable to the term *convulsion*, as some seizures have no abnormal convulsive movements. Seizures are common in the paediatric population, occurring in 5%–7% of children. The normal organised tonic-clonic seizure patterns seen in older infants and children are not seen in neonates. Seizure patterns in neonates include focal clonic, multi-focal jerks, apnoea eye blinking and jitteriness. In young children, febrile seizure (FS) is the most common cause of seizure occurring in 3%–4%, followed by epileptic seizure occurring in 1%. Epilepsy should not be diagnosed unless seizures are recurrent and unprovoked (e.g. by fever or hypoglycaemia). Epilepsy can be generalised (e.g. absence, myoclonic, tonic-clonic), focal (e.g. temporal lobe epilepsy) and epileptic spasms (e.g. infantile spasms). Seizures have to be differentiated from non-epileptic seizures (e.g. pseudo-seizure, breath-holding attacks) defined as motor activity or behaviour that resembles epileptic seizures but without abnormal/excessive discharges of neurones (EEG normal).

Possible Diagnoses

Infants	Children
Common	
HIE	Febrile seizure
Cerebral haemorrhage	Epilepsy (generalised and focal)
Metabolic (e.g. hypoglycaemia, hypocalcaemia)	Metabolic (e.g. hypoglycaemia)
Infection (e.g. meningitis)	Infection (encephalitis)
Developmental/malformation	Non-epileptic seizures (pseudo-seizure)
Neonatal epilepsy syndromes	
Neonatal withdrawal syndrome	
Rare	
Fifth-day seizure (benign idiopathic neonatal seizure)	Cerebral haemorrhage
Inborn errors of metabolism	Intracranial tumours
Mitochondrial disease	Drug induced
Pyridoxine dependent	Menkes kinky-hair disease

Differential Diagnosis at a Glance

	Febrile Seizure	Epilepsy	Metabolic	Infection	Pseudo-Seizure
Positive family history	Possible	Possible	No	No	No
Previous episode	Possible	Yes	Possible	No	Possible
Associated fever	Yes	No	No	Yes	No
Age younger than 5 years	Yes	Possible	Yes	Yes	No
Usually generalised	Yes	Possible	Yes	Possible	Yes

Recommended Investigations

***   Blood: FBC, CRP, blood culture, electrolytes, glucose, calcium, magnesium, urea
***   Prolactin blood level if pseudo-seizure is suspected (high in genuine seizure)

*** EEG for afebrile seizures

*** Neuroimaging for suspected encephalitis, abscess, focal seizures, complex partial seizures and increased intracranial pressure

Top Tips

- Seizures occur during the neonatal period more than at any other period in children because of the high incidence of infections, trauma to the brain, structural lesions of the brain and metabolic disorders. HIE is the most common cause of neonatal seizures.
- In neonatal seizures, subsequent developmental delay, cerebral palsy, epilepsy and death are related to low Apgar scores at 5 minutes.
- FS is a benign condition provoked by sudden rise of fever. Investigation in an otherwise healthy child is unnecessary except for urine examination.
- The minimum workup metabolic screen in neonates includes serum amino acids, urine organic acids and blood lactate for mitochondrial disease. For the first unprovoked seizure in an otherwise healthy child, include blood tests for glucose, calcium, magnesium, electrolytes and urea, and an EEG.
- Prolonged seizure, unresponsiveness to anti-epileptic drugs (AEDs), and the need for more than one AED to control the seizure are poor prognostic features in any seizure type.
- Hypomagnesaemia (magnesium <1.5 mg/dL) is very often associated with hypocalcaemia. The seizure will not respond to calcium but intramuscular injection of magnesium will correct both conditions.
- Seizures occurring during the initial phase of sleep or on waking in an older child are suggestive of benign partial epilepsy (Rolandic) (10%–15% of all childhood epilepsy) or juvenile myoclonic epilepsy (5%–10% of all childhood epilepsy).
- Pseudo-seizure can sometimes be difficult to differentiate from epileptic seizure: video recording and serum prolactin (increased in true epilepsy) can help.

Red Flags

- Neonatal seizures may be the only sign of CNS structural abnormality, including malformation. Their recognition is critical as presentation is often subtle (such as oral-lingual movements).
- FS should be differentiated from meningitis; children with CNS infection were usually unwell with headache, vomiting and lethargy before the onset of the seizure, with more persistent post-ictal impaired or loss of consciousness.
- Remember that epilepsy is more than just a seizure. It is associated with significant co-morbidities, including learning disability, anxiety and depression. Children are at risk for early mortality and sudden unexplained death in epilepsy.
- Medication noncompliance is an important cause of status epilepticus. Children with epilepsy should adhere to the prescribed medication regimen.
- Focal seizures are often more serious than generalised seizures. Focal seizures can be the presenting features of herpes encephalitis or cerebral tumours. Timely neuroimaging is essential.

FURTHER READING

Pavone P, Corsello G, Ruggieri M et al. Benign and severe early-life seizures: A round in the first year of life. *Ital J Pediatr* 2018;44:54.

Stafstrom CE, Carmant L. Seizures and epilepsy: An overview for neuroscientists. *Cold Spring Harb Perspective Med* 2015;5(6):a022426.

SLEEP DISORDERS

Clinician Overview

Children require sufficient sleep, but the amount required as sufficient varies. Young infants need on average 14 hours of sleep per 24 hours, which is almost evenly distributed throughout the day and night due to incompletely developed circadian rhythm. Children aged 6–12 years require about 10–11 hours and teens about 9 hours. Insomnia is characterised by difficulty in initiating and/or maintaining sleep, waking too early or having restless sleep. It is fairly normal for infants to wake several times at night; some 30% of infants do this. Older children (4–12 years) commonly present with bedtime resistance. Insufficient sleep at night is likely to affect the child's mood and behaviour during the day, leading to school problems such as reduced attention span, aggressiveness and poor performance. Sleep-related breathing disorders include central sleep apnoea and obstructive sleep apnoea. Parasomnia is disruptive sleep-related disorders occurring during the non-rapid eye movement (NREM) sleep such as sleep-walking, sleep terrors and confusional arousal. Those disorders occurring during rapid eye movement (REM) sleep include absent sleep paralysis. Hypersomnia, or excessive sleep, includes narcolepsy.

Possible Diagnoses

Infants	Children
Common	
Any illness, any pain or discomfort	Insomnia for any illness, pain or itching
Obstructive sleep apnoea (OSA)	Sleep-related breathing disorders
Drugs	Parasomnia (e.g. nightmares)
Normal sleep patterns	Hypersomnia (e.g. narcolepsy)
	Sleep-related epilepsies
Rare	
Pierre Robin sequence	Sleep-related movement disorders
Congenital hypoventilation syndrome	Side effects of drugs (methylphenidate), caffeine
	Kleine–Levin syndrome (KLS)
	Sleeping sickness (African trypanosomiasis)
	Central sleep apnoea

Differential Diagnosis at a Glance

	Insomnias	Breathing-Disorders	Parasomnia	Hypersomnia	Sleep-Related Epilepsies
Mostly in infants	Yes	Possible	No	No	No
Excessive movements	Yes	Possible	Yes	No	Yes
Disruptive sleep	Yes	Yes	Yes	No	Possible
Long daytime sleep	Possible	Possible	Possible	Yes	No
EEG diagnostic	No	No	No	No	Yes

Recommended Investigations

In the vast majority of cases, investigations are unlikely to be required.

** Polysomnography with oxygen saturation monitoring is very useful for insomnia evaluation, such as OSA, narcolepsy and nocturnal seizures

** HLA *DQB1*06,02* can be a useful marker in patients with narcolepsy and cataplexy

Top Tips

- Small infants often have apnoea episodes at night, which are harmless, lasting usually less than 10 seconds, and are not associated with cyanosis, decreased oxygen saturation or bradycardia.
- Nightmares are differentiated from night terrors by easy recall of the event. Night terrors are usually associated with a cry or piercing scream; the child looks flushed, frightened and agitated, and is not easily aroused. The child cannot recall the event the next morning.
- OSA, which manifests as snoring and frequent cessation of sleep, is an important cause of insomnia. Children with Down's syndrome, triangular chin and long soft palate are at risk of having OSA. The child may need tonsillectomy and/or adenoidectomy.
- During sleepwalking, parents should not try to waken or restrain the child. Telling the child about the event is unnecessary. If episodes are frequent, scheduled waking may help: the child is gently and briefly woken 15–30 minutes before the episode is due, and this is repeated for a month.
- Narcolepsy is characterised by recurring daytime sleepiness, often associated with disrupted sleep at night, cataplexy (loss of muscle control when, for example, laughing), sleep paralysis and hypnagogic phenomenon (auditory or visual illusion or hallucination when falling asleep).
- In contrast to narcolepsy, Kleine–Levin syndrome is rare. It is characterised by long and recurrent hypersomnia, hyperphagia and sometimes hypersexuality.
- Although many parents and clinicians often turn to medication to treat child insomnia, it is far more important to search for any underlying cause (e.g. anxiety) that needs to be treated first.

Red Flags

- Children with narcolepsy may not only present with daytime sleepiness but also with behaviour problems, irritability and deterioration of school performance.
- Narcolepsy is a lifelong problem. Although the tricyclic antidepressant clomipramine remains the main treatment, remember that it may cause numerous and unpleasant side effects: constipation, urinary retention and dry mouth.
- Sleepwalking occurs occasionally in 20%–40% and frequently in 3%–4%. The typical age is 4–8 years. Serious accidents may occur; securing the home (e.g. windows, locked doors) is essential.
- Beware of several sleep-related epileptic seizures: benign partial epilepsy with centrotemporal spikes (rolanic), benign epilepsy with affective symptoms, benign occipital epilepsy and Panayiotopoulos syndrome. Autonomic symptoms and secondary generalisation may occur in these sleep-related epilepsies.
- Be aware of nocturnal frontal lobe epilepsy (NFLE), which may mimic night terrors. A child with NFLE has a variety of motor features (kicking, hitting, thrashing, cycling and scissoring of the legs) and vocalisation (shouting, grunting, screaming and coughing). EEG may help in establishing diagnosis.

FURTHER READING

El-Shakankiry HM. Sleep physiology and sleep diseases in children. *Nat Sci Sleep* 2011;3:101–114.
Jarrin DC, McGrath JJ, Drake CL. Beyond sleep duration: Distinct sleep dimensions are associated with obesity in children and adolescents. *Int J Obes (Lond)* 2013;37(4):552–558.
Thorpy MJ. Classification of sleep disorders. *Neurotherapeutics* 2012;9(4):687–701.

TREMOR

Clinical Overview

Hyperkinetic movements are involuntary and excess movements that include dystonia, chorea, athetosis, myoclonia, tics and tremor. Of these, tremor is the most common type in children, which is a rhythmic, involuntary oscillation of part of the body, usually the hands, neck or head (titubation). It is classified as rest tremor (e.g. Parkinson's disease or drug induced), which is noted when the hands are resting on the lap, and the more common action tremor, which is produced by voluntary muscle contraction. Action tremor is either postural when affected arms are extended in front of the body (e.g. physiological or essential tremor) or target-directed movement such as intention (e.g. cerebellar tremor). Tremor is absent during sleep. It may be associated with serious neurological or metabolic disease. Tremor needs to be differentiated from tics and chorea.

Possible Diagnoses

Infants	Children
Common	
Normal jitteriness/tremor	Physiological tremor
Infants of maternal addiction	Essential tremor (ET)
Seizure (e.g. hypoglycaemia)	Psychogenic
Infantile tremor syndrome	Medications (e.g. β-2 agonists for asthma)
Cerebral irritation	Cerebellar tremor
Rare	
	Ataxic cerebral palsy
	Wilson's disease
	Acute confusional state
	Writing tremor
	Fragile X–associated tremor
	Pheochromocytoma
	Hyperthyroidism
	Cerebello-thalamo-cortical tremor
	Juvenile Parkinson's disease
	Autosomal dominant familial cortical myoclonic tremor
	Acute intermittent porphyria

Differential Diagnosis at a Glance

	Physiological	Essential	Psychogenic	Medications	Cerebellar
Positive family history	No	Yes	No	No	No
Present at rest	Possible	No	Yes	Yes	No
Progressive	No	Yes	Possible	No	Yes
Associated ataxia	No	No	No	Possible	Yes

Recommended Investigations

*** Urine copper and serum ceruloplasmin in suspected cases of Wilson's disease
*** Urine for toxicology from a neonate, and if possible from the mother

*** Thyroid function tests for suspected hyperthyroidism
*** Imaging of the brain for cerebral or cerebellar causes

Top Tips

- Children with unexplained hepatitis should be screened for Wilson's disease.
- Common benign neonatal non-epileptic movements include tremor (jitteriness) and sleep myoclonia. Tremor, a rhythmic involuntary movement of equal amplitude, is common in healthy neonates, occurring in up to two-thirds during the first 3 days of life.
- Drug addiction (e.g. cocaine, heroin, amphetamine) among pregnant women has increased steadily over the years. The result is an increased incidence of neonatal withdrawal syndrome with irritability, jitteriness and occasionally seizures. A detailed maternal drug history is essential.
- Physiological tremor is a fine tremor and rarely visible to the eye. It occurs in most individuals when the arms are extended. Tremor is enhanced by anxiety, stress or caffeine intake. More subtle tremor can be demonstrated by holding a piece of paper in outstretched hands.
- ET is the most common type of tremor: autosomal dominant (30%–60%), typically slowly progressive, symmetrically bilateral and significantly worsening during action like handwriting and spiral drawing.
- Tremor needs to be differentiated from tics, which are actually jerks, non-rhythmic and can affect any muscle; tics can be temporarily suppressed. Chorea is non-rhythmic, irregular, more rapid than tremor, jerky and predominately affects the face.
- Drugs causing tremor include amphetamine, asthma medications such as β-2 agonist and theophylline, lithium, anticonvulsants such as valproate, and tricyclic antidepressants. Of these, the β-2 agonist salbutamol is by far the most common drug causing tremor and tachycardia. Although these are benign, parents should be made aware of these side effects.

Red Flags

- Neonatal tremor/jitteriness is frequently misdiagnosed as seizure resulting in unnecessary investigations and treatment with anticonvulsants. This tremor has no abnormal gaze or eye movement, cyanosis, bradycardia or tachycardia; it is provoked by stretching a joint and stops on holding the limb.
- Any neonatal tremor may be due to prenatal exposure to maternal marijuana or neonatal withdrawal effect from other narcotic use. It often persists for 30 days. History taking is essential.
- Essential tremor is often confused with cerebellar tremor as both worsen with action. Cerebellar tremor is typically intentional and is associated with ataxia and other cerebellar signs.
- In any child with progressive or acute tremor, serious conditions such as Wilson's disease, hyperthyroidism, hypoglycaemia, hypocalcaemia, neuroblastoma and pheochromocytoma have to be excluded.

FURTHER READING

Huntsman RJ, Lowry NJ, Sankaran K. Non-epileptic motor phenomena in the neonate. *Paediatr Child Health* 2008;13(8):680–684.

13 ENDOCRINE

DELAYED PUBERTY

Clinical Overview

Puberty begins with the secretion of the pituitary gonadotropins, follicle-stimulating hormone (FSH) and luteinising hormone (LH), which stimulate sex steroids testosterone and eostradiol to induce the appearance of secondary sexual characteristics. Breast bud appears in females between 8 and 13 years. Menarche occurs at the median age of 13 years, 2–3 years after the appearance of breast bud. Penile and scrotal enlargement usually occurs 1 year after the testicular enlargement over 4 mL. Delayed puberty (DP) is defined as a delay of pubertal changes (absence of breast bud) beyond 13 years in girls or incompletion of puberty within 5 years from the occurrence of breast bud. In males, DP is defined as testes <4 mL aged 14 years, or an absence of secondary sexual signs by the age of 16 years, or incompletion of puberty within 5 years from its start. The cause of DP in the vast majority of boys and in most girls is constitutional, which is usually associated with delayed growth and skeletal maturation and positive history in the parents. The exceptions to that are boys with Klinefelter's syndrome (XXO gonadal dysgenesis), who are tall with long arms and legs, having normal adrenarche but small testes.

Possible Diagnoses

Infants	Children
Common	
Not applicable	Constitutional
	Functional hypo-gonadotropic hypogonadism (FHH)
	Structural hypo-gonadotropic hypogonadism (SHH)
	Intensive physical exercise
	Gonadal failure (Turner's, Noonan's syndromes)
Rare	
	Central nervous system (CNS) tumour (craniopharyngioma)
	Prader-Willi syndrome
	Hyperprolactinaemia
	Laurence–Moon–Biedl syndrome
	Irradiation of the gonads, chemotherapy
	Following bone marrow transplantation
	Testicular feminisation syndrome
	Chronic psychiatric disorders
	Klinefelter's syndrome

Differential Diagnosis at a Glance

	Constitutional	FHH	SHH	Intense Physical	Gonadal Failure
Otherwise healthy	Yes	No	No	Yes	Possible
Short stature	Yes	Possible	Yes	No	Yes
Positive family history	Yes	No	No	No	No
Delayed bone age	Yes	Possible	Yes	No	Possible
FSH, LH levels	Yes	Possible	Yes	Possible	No

Recommended Investigations

- *** Full blood count (FBC), C-reactive protein (CRP): anaemia with high CRP suggests Crohn's disease
- *** Screening blood tests for coeliac disease
- *** Hormonal assay: levels of FSH/LH, gonadotropin-releasing hormone
- *** Thyroid function tests for suspected thyroid disorders
- *** Chromosomal analysis for suspected cases of Turner's (X0) and Klinefelter's (XXY) syndromes
- *** Wrist X-ray for bone age
- *** Pelvic ultrasound scan to detect ovarian cysts or tumour; testicular ultrasound for tumour
- *** Radiological investigation for suspected case of Crohn's disease
- *** Cranial MRI of the head for hypo-gonadotropic hypogonadism to exclude CNS pathologies

Top Tips

- When using the Tanner growth chart for pubertal stages in a child with DP, the heights of the parents and siblings should be obtained.
- Children with constitutional DP can be reassured. This is a normal variant of puberty timing with good outcome for final height and future reproductive capacity.
- Puberty can be assessed by bone age (wrist X-ray): if bone age is within 1 year of the child's age, puberty has not or has only just started; bone age within 2 years indicates the child is in puberty.
- A case of a very thin child with DP suggests the possibility of anorexia nervosa or excessive sport activity, while obesity may suggest Prader-Willi or Laurence–Moon–Biedl syndrome.
- In girls with DP and short stature, Turner's syndrome should be considered. Pelvic ultrasound scan and chromosomal analysis should be carried out. High levels of FSH and LH are found.
- Remember that girls with Turner's syndrome achieve normal adrenarche and axillary hair at appropriate age. They do not develop menstruation.
- Hormonal treatment is often indicated in boys in constitutional DP (with oxandrolone aged 11.5 years and testosterone aged over 13.5 years) and in girls (with ethinylestradiol or oestrogens) if the DP and/or growth are causing distress or school underperformance.

Red Flags

- While the principal cause of DP in boys is constitutional, girls have more frequent pathological causes, e.g. anorexia nervosa, chronic diseases, intensive exercise or chromosomal abnormalities.
- Constitutional DP is a diagnosis of exclusion; therefore, alternative causes should be considered, including functional HH causing transient DP (e.g. malabsorption, renal insufficiency, anorexia), structural HH causing permanent DP (CNS pathologies) and gonadal failure in both sexes.
- Beware that chronic diseases (e.g. Crohn's and coeliac diseases) may initially present as DP.
- All girls with an inguinal hernia should undergo a pelvic ultrasound scan examination before the operation to exclude testicular feminisation (currently termed androgen insensitivity syndrome).
- In girls with otherwise normal sexual maturation but delayed menarche and galactorrhoea, prolactinoma is likely. Urgent prolactin level and MRI of the brain should be considered.

FURTHER READING

Bozzola M, Bozzola E, Montalbano C et al. Delayed puberty versus hypogonadism: A challenge for the pediatricians. *Ann Pediatr Endocrinol Metab* 2018;23(2):57–61.

HEIGHT, EXCESSIVE (TALL STATURE)

Clinical Overview

Growth is influenced by many factors such as hereditary, genetic, illness, nutritional, medication, hormonal and psychological influences. Tall stature is defined as a height of more than 2.0 standard deviations or a height above the 97th centile for age and sex. The condition is a less common reason for concern and referral to specialist than short stature. As a general rule, a child's potential height ranges between the averages of the parents' heights. Tall parents usually have tall children. The incidence of pathology in cases of tall stature is very low (around 1%–2%). Although growth hormone (GH) is known to be responsible for gigantism and acromegaly, other conditions associated with an excessive GH secretion and possible gigantism include McCune–Albright syndrome (incidence of gigantism 15%–20%).

Possible Diagnoses

Infants	Children
Common	
Hereditary/genetic	Hereditary/genetic
Hyperinsulinism	Constitutional
Large-of-date babies	Klinefelter's syndrome (chromosome: 47, XXY)
Infant of diabetic mother	Obesity
Overweight	Precocious puberty (McCune–Albright syndrome)
	Marfan's syndrome
Rare	
Sotos' syndrome	Pituitary Gigantism
Beckwith–Wiedemann syndrome	Sotos' syndrome
	Beckwith–Wiedemann syndrome
	Homocystinuria
	Hypogonadism
	Neurofibromatosis
	Hyperthyroidism
	Proteus syndrome
	Congenital generalised lipodystrophy

Differential Diagnosis at a Glance

	Familial	Constitutional	Klinefelter's Syndrome	Obesity	Precocious Puberty
Tall parents	Yes	Possible	No	Possible	No
Normal physical examination	Yes	Yes	No	No	No
Normal linear growth rate	Yes	No	No	No	No
Comorbidity	No	No	Yes	Yes	Yes
Advanced bone age	No	Yes	No	Yes	Yes

Recommended Investigations

*** Urine for homocystine
*** Insulin-growth factor 1 and GH in blood: in cases of pituitary gigantism, acromegaly

** Plasma levels of FSH, LH for Klinefelter's syndrome
*** Karyotyping for suspected cases of Klinefelter's syndrome
*** Skeletal X-ray for a child with precocious puberty (e.g. McCune–Albright syndrome)
*** Echocardiography for Marfan's syndrome to exclude aneurysm
*** Cranial MRI for suspected pituitary tall stature to exclude adenoma

Top Tips

- Child's length or height must be measured accurately. In children younger than 24 months, recumbent length and standing height are not the same; the former being significantly greater. Measurement with tape is inaccurate.
- Girls are more likely than boys to be concerned early about their tall stature. Society perceives tall and slender girls as beautiful, but not those with excessive height.
- The most common cause of tall stature is familial or genetic (about 80%). Children are tall from early childhood, have tall parents, high normal growth rate and a bone age compatible with chronological age. Constitutional tall stature is associated with normal length at birth, early accelerated growth that slows down after the age of 4–5 years and slightly or moderately advanced bone age.
- Over 50% of obese children have a height in the 70%–99% range on the centile chart.
- Although treatment with oestrogen in tall girls and androgen in tall boys may be effective, this is associated with numerous side effects, and is controversial. Epiphysiodesis for predicted adult height of >205 cm in boys and >185 in girls should be considered.

Red Flags

- Beware that some tall children, especially girls, may be teased and ridiculed leading to psychiatric problems such as anxiety, depression and social withdrawal. They are also at risk of developing orthopaedic problems, e.g. kyphosis and scoliosis.
- One important cause of tall stature is precocious puberty occurring simultaneously with premature sexual development. The skin should be examined for café-au-lait maculae to exclude McCune–Albright syndrome, which is also associated with bone fibrous dysplasia.
- Be aware that children with Klinefelter's syndrome often present with complaints other than height, e.g. gynaecomastia, behaviour problems such as aggressiveness, excessive shyness and antisocial acts such as fire setting and crimes.
- Children with Marfan's syndrome are at risk of early death because of progressive aortic dilatation and rupture. Arachnodactyly and lens dislocation are important clues that need to be differentiated from homocystinuria that is associated with developmental delay.

FURTHER READING

Stalman SE, Pons A, Wit JM et al. Diagnostic work-up and follow-up children with tall stature: A simplified algorithm for clinical practice. *J Clin Res Pediatr Endocrinol* 2015;7(4):260–267.

PRECOCIOUS PUBERTY

Clinical Overview

Normal sexual development begins in girls with breast development, followed by the appearance of pubic hair (sometimes simultaneously with breast development), axillary hair, onset of menstruation, acne and adult body odour. In boys, it begins with testicular enlargement followed by enlargement of the penis, the appearance of pubic hair, deepening of the voice, acne and adult body odour. Precocious puberty (PP) is defined as puberty occurring at an unusual age, i.e. before the age of 8 years in girls or before 9 years in boys. Puberty nowadays starts earlier than in previous generations. Puberty depends on increased production of kisspeptin in the hypothalamus resulting in increased gonadotropin-releasing hormone (GnRH), which acts on the pituitary to release the gonadotropins LH and FSH, which stimulate sex hormone production by the gonads. The causes of PP are best divided into gonadotropin-dependent central (idiopathic or with identifiable causes), gonadotropin-independent (adrenal and gonadal causes) or partial PP (thelarche, adrenarche, menarche). In more than 90% of girls and 50% of boys, the cause of PP is idiopathic, i.e. no identifiable cause. The main differentiating feature between central (hypothalamic) and adrenal causes is that the PP is always isosexual in the former and testes remain small in the latter cause.

Possible Diagnoses

Infants	Children
Common	
CNS injury	Partial (incomplete) precocious puberty (PPP)
Adrenal (e.g. congenital adrenal)	Central idiopathic precocious puberty
Ovarian (e.g. McCune–Albright)	Central with identifiable causes (e.g. hamartoma)
Iatrogenic (external sex hormones)	Gonads (ovarian cysts, McCune–Albright syndrome)
PPP (e.g. premature thelarche)	Adrenal (e.g. congenital adrenal hyperplasia, tumour)
Rare	
	Iatrogenic (external sources of sex hormones)
	Irradiation of the brain
	Familial PP in males
	Teratoma (e.g. in the mediastinum)

Differential Diagnosis at a Glance

	PPP	Idiopathic Central PP	Central PP with a Cause	Gonad-Causing PP	Adrenal Causing PP
Normal growth	Yes	No	No	No	No
Gonadotropin dependent	No	Yes	Yes	No	No
More in girls than in boys	Yes	Yes	No	No	No
Advanced bone age	No	Yes	Yes	Yes	Yes
High FSH+LH	No	Yes	Yes	No	No

Recommended Investigations

*** Hormonal assay of GnRH, LH, FSH

*** GnRH stimulation test (in central PP, the LH and FSH levels are increased)

*** Serum level of I7-hydroxyprogesterone, dehydroepiandrosterone, cortisol and aldosterone in cases of congenital adrenal hyperplasia (CAH)

*** Wrist X-ray to assess bone maturation

*** Pelvic ultrasound scan and adrenal visualisation for CAH

*** Computed tomography scan or MRI of the head for all cases suspected of central causes of PP

** Skeletal survey for bony fibrous dysplasia for a child with PP and hyperpigmented spots

Top Tips

- Puberty can easily be assessed by bone age: if bone age is within 1 year of chronological age, puberty either has not or has just started; bone age within 2 years indicates the child is in puberty.
- Isolated thelarche is characterised by normal growth, age-appropriate skeletal maturation, pre-pubertal uterus and ovaries and isolated FSH elevation with pre-pubertal LH level.
- PPP is either an isolated breast development (precocious thelarche) or sexual hair appearance (precocious adrenarche) without other signs of puberty occurring before the age of 8 years in girls and 9 years in boys. PPP is usually benign and non-progressive. Onset younger than 3 years is frequently associated with regression over 1–3 years; later onset usually progresses slowly as PP.
- In precocious thelarche, the nipple is characteristically pale, immature, thin and transparent. In PP the nipple is mature and prominent with dark areolas indicating high circulating oestrogen.
- PP may have adverse effects on social behaviour and psychological development. Early growth spurt causes rapid bone maturation, resulting in early epiphyseal fusion and short stature.
- Low-dose radiation of the brain may induce PP in girls; high-dose radiation may induce PP in both sexes.
- Hypothyroidism can cause PP; children are, however, short and the growth velocity is decreased.
- Growth acceleration and advanced bone age (wrist X-ray) favour true PP against PPP.

Red Flags

- In any child with PP, careful search of the skin is essential: café-au-lait maculae with smooth borders suggest NF-1; larger café-au-lait patches with irregular outlines are consistent with the McCune–Albright syndrome (polyostotic fibrous dysplasia of bone, and ovarian cysts).
- Be aware that children with hypothalamic lesion may present with diabetes insipidus (polydipsia, polyuria), hyperthermia, obesity or loss of weight, or inappropriate crying or laughter.
- PP may put girls at risk of sexual abuse and psychological trauma from teasing and bullying.
- A child with precocious thelarche or adrenarche still needs careful evaluation, as these cannot often be easily and definitely differentiated from true PP.
- Full investigation, including imaging of the CNS and abdomen, should be carried out for all children with PP who have progressive signs of puberty, are younger than 8 years, with neurological signs or if the diagnosis is uncertain.
- Hypothalamic hamartoma (ectopic tissue secreting pulse GnRH) is the most common identifiable lesion causing PP. Examination of visual acuity, visual fields and eye fundi is essential.

FURTHER READING

Bajpal A, Menon PSN. Contemporary issues in precocious puberty. *Indian Endocrinol Metabol* 2011;15 (Suppl 3):S172–S179.

Stephen MD, Zage PE, Waguespack SG. Gonadotropin-dependent precocious puberty: Neoplastic causes. *Int J Pediatr Endocrinol* 2011;2011(1):184502.

SHORT STATURE

Clinical Overview

Human growth is a complex physiological process regulated by genetic, hormonal, nutritional, environmental and psychological factors. About 80% of the variation in height is determined genetically. Short stature is defined as height under 2.0 standard deviations below the mean or under the third percentile. The three most common causes of short stature worldwide are familial, constitutional delay and malnutrition. Familial short stature is seen in normal children who have short parents, normal growth rate and bone age, and enter puberty at the normal time. Their ultimate height is related to their parental height. Children with constitutional delay have a normal growth rate, but delayed onset of puberty and bone age. Because of delayed bone age, they have more time to grow; they usually achieve a normal adult height appropriate to the family pattern. Chronic diseases causing short stature are mainly due to malnutrition.

Possible Diagnoses

Infants	Children
Common	
Intrauterine growth retardation	Familial short stature
Skeletal abnormalities	Constitutional delay
Malnutrition	Malnutrition
Emotional deprivation	Chronic disease (e.g. chronic renal disease)
	Chromosomal (e.g. Turner's syndrome)
Rare	
	Idiopathic short stature
	Endocrine (e.g. hypothyroidism, poorly controlled diabetes)
	Emotional deprivation
	Skeletal abnormality (hypochondroplasia)
	Congenital heart diseases
	PP
	Chronic anaemia
	Survivors of cancer
	Chronic diseases (coeliac disease, Crohn's disease)

Differential Diagnosis at a Glance

	Familial Short Stature	Constitutional Short Stature	Malnutrition	Chronic Disease	Chromosomal
Normal height increase >5 cm/year	Yes	Yes	Possible	Possible	No
Short parents	Yes	Possible	Yes	No	No
Normal physical examination	Yes	Yes	No	No	No
Normal labor findings	Yes	Yes	No	No	No
Delayed bone age	No	Yes	Yes	Yes	No

Recommended Investigations

*** FBC: to exclude anemia
*** Blood glucose if growth hormone (GH) deficiency is suspected

*** Thyroid function test to confirm hypothyroidism
** GH check, often done by checking the IGF-1 (insulin-like growth factor-1)
*** Liver function tests, urea and electrolytes if liver or renal disease is suspected
*** Genetic studies, beginning with a karyotype for Turner's syndrome
*** Chromosomal microarray, whole exome sequencing, and hybridization testing
*** Bone age to differentiate familial short stature from constitutional delay
*** Ultrasonography of the heart, kidney and ovaries for Turner's syndrome

Top Tips

- The highest growth rate occurs in uterus (6 cm at 12 weeks' gestation to 50 cm at term) and from birth to 1 year of life (23–28 cm); decreasing aged 1–3 years (7.5–13 cm) and aged 3 years to puberty (5–7 cm); but increasing at puberty (8–9 cm in girls and 10–10.5 cm in boys).
- Children's growth is like tree growth: they grow faster in spring and summer; therefore, growth velocity should be measured for 1 year.
- When children present with short stature, doctors need to determine whether they require extensive evaluation (e.g. hormonal, chromosomal) or conservative monitoring for children with idiopathic short stature that includes familial short stature and constitutional delay of growth.
- GH is a major counter-regulatory hormone to insulin; therefore, children with GH deficiency may present with hypoglycaemia, particularly during fasting or mild illness.
- Measuring the height of both parents is essential in evaluating a child with short stature. It helps diagnose familial short stature and predict the ultimate height of the children.
- Short stature is often confused with growth failure. Short stature is defined as height under the third percentile with normal annual growth rate, while growth failure is defined as a growth rate of <5 cm.
- Parents of children with short stature often seek medical services because of a possible 'endocrine' cause; endocrine diseases are rare and no more than 5% of causes.

Red Flags

- When evaluating children with short stature, it is more important how their growth rate has been rather than where the percentile is on the chart.
- Remember that the vast majority of short children do not have GH deficiency, but because the deficiency is potentially treatable, it must be considered carefully and excluded.
- Always consider Turner's syndrome when pubertal delay is combined with short stature. Children with Turner's syndrome may have hypertension and cardiovascular and renal malformation.
- Children with chronic renal disease, who are receiving dialysis or transplant, commonly have poor linear growth, which is a high risk factor of poor school performance, frequent hospitalisations and death.
- Short stature can be more a social than a clinical problem, being often a source of ridicule and torment, teasing and bullying at school. Teaching patients how to respond assertively and effectively to bullying and teasing to ensure preserving self-esteem and confidence is essential.

FURTHER READING

Jee YH, Baron J. The biology of stature. *J Pediatr* 2016;173:32–38.
Ku E, Fine RN, Hsu CY et al. Height at first RRT and mortality in children. *Clin J Am Soc Nephrol* 2016;11(5):832–839.

14 SKIN

ANAEMIA AND PALLOR

Clinical Overview

Normal skin colour is mostly determined by the child's constitutional degree of melanin content of the skin resulting from hereditary and racial backgrounds. Pallor or reduced or loss of the colour of skin or mucous membrane can be caused by a variety of conditions including normal complexion, lack of exposure to sunlight, anaemia, emotional stress, shock or chronic disease (Figure 14.1). Unless pallor is accompanied by clinical signs of anaemia (pallor of the palmar, lip, mouth, conjunctiva and nail bed), it is of no great significance. If these sites appear pale, haemoglobin (Hb) needs to be checked to exclude anaemia. Anaemia is the most common nutritional deficiency worldwide; around 2 billion people (around 30% of world's population) are anaemic. It is defined as an Hb level of less than 11 g/dL. A detailed account of anaemia is beyond the scope of this book.

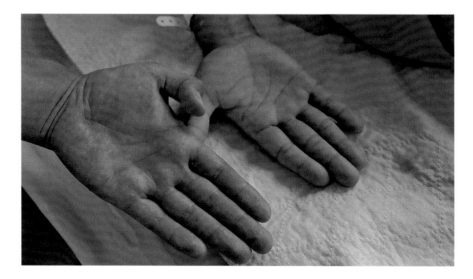

FIGURE 14.1   Pallor in the hand of the patient on the right.

Possible Diagnoses

Infants	Children
Common	
Feto-fetal transfusion	Iron-deficiency anaemia (IDA)
Blood loss	Thalassaemia
Haemolytic anaemia	Chronic disease (infection, inflammation, tumour)
Infection	Haemolytic anaemia (e.g. spherocytosis)
Physiological anaemia	Haemoglobinopathy (e.g. sickle cell anaemia [SCA])

(Continued)

(Continued)

Infants	Children
Rare	
Disseminated intravascular coagulation (DIC)	Lead poisoning
Osteopetrosis	Drugs
Red cell aplasia	Haemolytic uraemic syndrome
	Inflammatory bowel disease (e.g. Crohn's disease [CD])
	Aplastic anaemia
	Hypothyroidism
	Storage disease
	Megaloblastic anaemia (folic acid and vitamin B_{12} deficiency)
	Coeliac disease

Differential Diagnosis at a Glance

	IDA	Thalassaemia	Chronic Disease	Haemolytic Anemia	Haemoglobinopathy
Splenomegaly	Possible	Yes	No	Yes	Yes
Reticulocytosis	No	Yes	No	Yes	Yes
Low ferritin	Yes	No	Possible	No	No
Decreased mean cell volume (MCV), mean corpuscular haemoglobin (MCH)	Yes	Yes	Possible	No	No
Jaundice	No	Yes	No	Yes	Yes

Recommended Investigations

*** Full blood count (FBC): Hb <11 g/dL is anaemia; MCV<70 fL) and MCH<26pg: microcytic hypochromic anaemia

*** Serum ferritin low in IDA

*** Liver function test (LFT): hyperbilirubinaemia suggestive of acute or chronic haemolysis

*** Reticulocyte count: high in haemolytic anaemia and in response to iron treatment

*** Vitamin B_{12} and folate (MCV >90) to exclude causes of megaloblastic anaemia

*** Hb-electrophoresis: HbS in SCA; high level of HbF to confirm thalassaemia

** Bone marrow examination is required to exclude other disorders such as aplastic anaemia

** Serum iron and iron binding capacity

Top Tips

- High Hb and RBCs in neonates are due to active erythropoiesis in response to low arterial oxygen saturation (AOS) during foetal life. This erythropoiesis ceases abruptly with the rise of AOS at birth. Low erythropoiesis continues for 6–10 weeks, causing a low Hb of 9–11 g/dL in full-term (physiological anaemia of infancy) and 7–9 g/dL in premature infants. This is the best stimulus for erythropoiesis and should not be suppressed by blood transfusion.

- By far the most common cause of anaemia is nutritional iron deficiency, which can be easily diagnosed by low MCV, MCH, and ferritin level. IDA is associated with suppressed immune and cognitive functions, slower growth, and poor motor and mental development.

- It can be difficult to exclude thalassaemia minor from IDA; both have low MCV and MCH. Ferritin can differentiate (normal or high in thalassaemia). Remember that IDA can co-exist with thalassaemia; therefore, HbA_2 >3.4% is diagnostic of a thalassaemia trait.
- Treatment with oral iron should be given to all children with Hb <11 g/dL for 4–6 weeks. Hb needs to be checked to ensure recovery of the anaemia.

Red Flags

- Ignoring the need to investigate even mild anaemia is a mistake; its presence may indicate a serious underlying disorder.
- Anaemia with low MCV/MCH should not be treated with iron before thalassaemia is excluded.
- In districts or localities with a high rate of socio-economic deprivation, IDA is common, exerting a negative impact on a child's development. School-age children with IDA may have impaired concentration and activity which affect learning. Screening for anaemia is important.
- Be aware that children with Crohn's disease may present with anaemia alone; ask whether there have been abdominal pain and weight loss (these form the three features of this disease).
- Adding tonics, vitamins or trace metals to iron therapy is of no scientific value; therefore, parents should be educated about this point.
- Iron preparations are an important cause of accidental overdose. Parents should keep the medicine away from children, and should be told about common side effects of iron.

FURTHER READING

World Health Organization. Micronutrient deficiencies. www.who.int//nutrition/en

BLISTERS (VESICLES AND BULLAE)

Clinical Overview

Blister is the lay terminology for both vesicle (Figure 14.2) and bulla (Figure 14.3). While a vesicle is a fluid-filled raised cavity less than 1 cm in diameter, a bulla is greater than 1 cm in diameter. Vesicles may occur on the mucosa of the mouth; it is however unusual to see them intact because there is so much friction and trauma from eating and moving the tongue. Blister eruption can be caused by infection such as varicella, bullous impetigo, herpes simplex or hereditary blistering disorders such as epidermolysis bullosa. Other causes include external factors such as sunburn and contact dermatitis, or immune-mediated cutaneous diseases such as dermatitis herpetiformis, bullous pemphigoid and pemphigus.

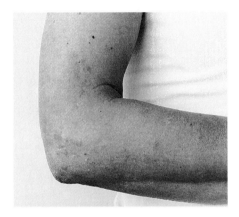

FIGURE 14.2   Vesicles.

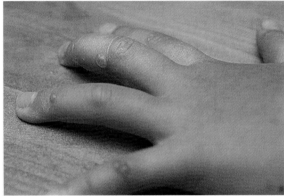

FIGURE 14.3   Bullae.

Possible Diagnoses

Infants	Children
Common	
Erythema toxicum neonatorum (ETN)	Chickenpox
Staphylococcal scalded skin syndrome	Urticaria
Herpes simplex virus	Atopic dermatitis (AD)
Herpetic gingivostomatitis	Erythema multiforme
Sucking blisters	Herpetic gingivostomatitis
Rare	
Scabies	Scabies
Epidermolysis bullosa	Eczema herpeticum
Epidermolytic hyperkeratosis	Hand-foot-mouth disease
Incontinentia pigmenti (first phase of the disease)	Porphyria
Toxic epidermal necrolysis (Lyell syndrome)	Stevens-Johnson syndrome
Neonatal pemphigus vulgaris	Drugs (e.g. naproxen)
Bullous Mastocytosis	Naproxen-induced pseudo-porphyria
Congenital syphilis	Contact dermatitis
Bullous pemphigoid of infancy	Dermatitis herpetiformis (DH)
	Bullous impetigo
	Pemphigus vulgaris
	Systemic lupus erythematosus (SLE)

Differential Diagnosis at a Glance

	Varicella	Urticaria	AD	Erythema Multiforme	Herpetic Gingivostomatitis
Bullae formation	No	Yes	No	Possible	No
With itching	Yes	Yes	Yes	Possible	No
Mucosal involvement	Yes	Possible	No	Yes	Yes
Fever	Yes	Possible	No	Possible	Yes
Chronic form	No	Yes	Yes	No	No

Recommended Investigations

** Blood for autoimmune antibodies and screening tests for coeliac disease

** Culture of swabs from the lesions of infected bullous impetigo to identify the infecting bacteria

** Biopsy of the lesions may be indicated for diagnosis of pemphigus or dermatitis herpetiformis

** PCR of vesicular fluid for the diagnosis of viral infections

Top Tips

• Note that the vesicles situated superficially are flaccid and rupture easily (e.g. bullous impetigo), whereas those arising from deeper layers are more tense.

• The Nikolsky sign (gentle rubbing produces similar skin lesions) is a useful test. This is positive in conditions like pemphigus or dermatitis herpetiformis (autoimmune blister diseases).

• ETN occurs in 15%–20% of neonates on the second day of life and regresses in 5–14 days. It is an inflammatory reaction of the skin characterised by papulo-vesicular and sterile pustules.

• Bullae at birth may be the first manifestation of epidermolysis bullosa. Bullae-caused staphylococci are usually not present at birth, and the bullae fluid appears infected in contrast to the clear uninfected fluid in epidermolysis bullosa.

• Hand-foot-mouth disease is a benign, common infection caused by the A16 strain of Coxsackie virus and arises usually first on the soft palate and tongue, followed by cutaneous lesions 1–2 days later.

• DH is an IgA-mediated chronic bullous disease characterised by intense itching and burning sensation. It is associated with coeliac disease, and both respond to a gluten-free diet.

• In contrast to adults, childhood herpes zoster is often not associated with localised pain or postherpetic neuralgia. Immunocompromised children may have severe zoster reaction.

• In an anaemic patient, a Mentzer index [MCV/RBC (millions)] <13 makes thalassaemia more likely that iron deficiency anaemia.

Red Flags

• Incising or puncturing bulla should not be performed as this may induce infection.

• Eczema herpeticum is a serious infection caused by herpes simplex virus, which is invading eczematous lesions. It can lead to death through dissemination of the virus to the brain and other organs or from secondary staphylococcal or streptococcal infection.

• Herpes simplex and varicella can become disseminated in immunocompromised patients. The child should be admitted and given appropriate treatment of intravenous acyclovir.

- Herpes zoster (shingles) is relatively benign except when it affects the ophthalmic division. Protection of the affected eye is essential.
- Scabies is a parasitic infestation caused by mites, with typical pruritic burrows found on the web spaces of the fingers. It is often misdiagnosed as eczema, prolonging the patient's suffering.
- Naproxen, a non-steroidal anti-inflammatory drug used as an inflammatory agent in rheumatic diseases, may cause an eruption characterised by erythema, vesicles and shallow atrophic scars after sun exposure.

FURTHER READING

Otten JV, Hashimoto T, Hertl M et al. Molecular diagnosis in autoimmune skin blistering conditions. *Curr Mol Med* 2014;14(1):69–95.

CYANOSIS

Clinical View

Cyanosis is caused by the presence of an excess of deoxygenated haemoglobin which is visible in the skin and mucous membranes (central cyanosis). The great majority of cyanotic children have either a pulmonary or a cardiac cause. Clinicians should be aware of cyanosis occurring in healthy normal children, for example peripheral cyanosis (acrocyanosis; Figure 14.4) noted in the vast majority of newly born babies (causing the Apgar score to be 9 instead of a complete 10) and in infants who are unwrapped and cold. Some healthy children may have perioral cyanosis in response to cold, with or without shivering, or following a rapid rise of fever. The causes of cardiac and pulmonary cyanosis are large and beyond the scope of this section.

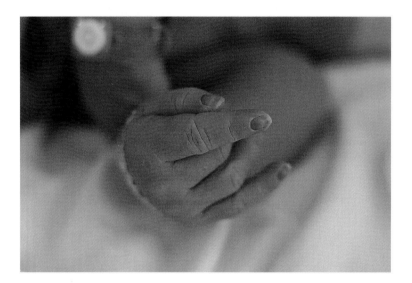

FIGURE 14.4   Cyanosis in a newborn.

Possible Diagnoses

Infants	Children
Common	
Acrocyanosis at birth	Breath-holding attacks (BHAs)
Respiratory distress syndrome (RDS)	Cardiac (failure, congenital heart disease [CHD])
Cyanotic CHD	Fever (onset with shivering)
Pulmonary hypertension	Pulmonary (pneumonia, severe asthma, pneumothorax)
Breath-holding attacks	Raynaud's phenomenon

(*Continued*)

(Continued)	
Infants	**Children**
Rare	
Shock and sepsis	Shock and sepsis (e.g. meningococcal infection)
Central hypoventilation	Neuromuscular disorders with respiratory or cardiac insufficiency
Methaemoglobinaemia (congenital)	Methaemoglobinaemia (ingestion of aniline dyes/nitrites)
High Hb (polycythaemia)	Foreign body
Neuromuscular diseases	Eisenmenger's syndrome
Pulmonary arteriovenous malformation	Arnold-Chiari malformation

Differential Diagnosis at a Glance

	BHA	Cardiac	Pulmonary	Fever	Raynaud's
Transient	Yes	No	Possible	Yes	Yes
Abolished by 100% oxygen	No	No	Yes	No	No
RDS signs (e.g. recession, grunting)	No	Possible	Yes	No	No
Low O_2 saturation	No	Yes	Yes	Possible	No
Peripheral	Possible	No	No	Possible	Yes

Recommended Investigations

** FBC to diagnose anaemia and polycythaemia; white blood cell count raised in bacterial infection

*** Blood gases: with breathing 100% oxygen a rapid improvement of the O_2 saturation in pulmonary arterial blood

*** Chest X-ray to differentiate pulmonary (e.g. infiltration) from cardiac causes (heart enlargement)

* Electrocardiogram (ECG) may show ventricular enlargement, arrhythmia or conduction defects

*** Echocardiography to provide the ultimate diagnosis

*** Lung function tests, including oxygen saturation by oximeter

Top Tips

- The three main signs of CHD are cyanosis, congestive cardiac failure and a heart murmur. The presence of central cyanosis in the newborn without respiratory distress favours CHD.
- Breathing 100% oxygen will help to differentiate between right-to-left (oxygen saturation remains low) and pulmonary or central hypoventilation.
- Increased Hb (polycythaemia) is more common in the newborns (e.g. following twin-to-twin transfusion, infants of diabetic mothers) than at any age later in childhood.
- Methaemoglobinaemia is either congenital due to autosomal inheritance (deficiency of the enzyme cytochrome reductase) or acquired by the ingestion of aniline dyes or nitrates. The cardinal presentation is cyanosis in an otherwise healthy child, not in distress and with normal physical examination. Cyanosis is reversed by giving vitamin C.
- Myocarditis is often caused by viral infection, and parvovirus B19, human herpes virus and enteroviruses are the main causes. Presentation is fever, myalgia, palpitation and syncope.

- Note that when a child manifests with blue lower extremities and pink upper extremities (differential cyanosis), the child has right-to-left shunt across a ductus arteriosus in the presence of coarctation or interrupted aortic arch.

Red Flags

- Mild cyanosis may escape detection if only the skin is examined. It is best detected by examining the nail beds, lips, tongue and mucous membranes.
- A newborn with cyanosis suspected of CHD, should have a prostaglandin infusion before arranging transportation to a cardiac unit to prevent closure of the ductus arteriosus.
- Differentiating cyanotic BHA from epilepsy can be challenging: The onset of BHA begins with crying, then apnoea, followed by facial cyanosis, limping and possible seizure. In epileptic seizure, children first have a seizure, then become blue.
- A child who becomes suddenly breathless, choking with or without cyanosis should be suspected of inhaling a foreign body. Every clinician should be knowledgeable in the management of eliminating it.
- In an asthmatic child who becomes suddenly cyanosed and breathless, pneumothorax must be ruled out.

FURTHER READING

Catto AG, Zgaga L, Theodoratou E et al. An evaluation of oxygen systems for treatment of childhood pneumonia. *BMC Public Health* 2011;11(Suppl 3):S28.

HYPER- AND HYPOPIGMENTED LESIONS

Clinical Overview

Pigmentary disorders are a common presentation to family physicians, paediatricians and dermatologists. Melanin (black) plays key roles in determining human skin colour. Other pigmentary determinants include haemoglobin (red), haemosiderin (brown) and carotene and bilirubin (yellow). In some cases, pigmentation is an external sign of a serious underlying systemic disorder. In general, multiple or generalised hyperpigmented lesions are associated with more serious underlying diseases than those with isolated lesions. Increased pigmentation (hyperpigmentation) may be caused by increased melanin production or increased number of melanocytes. It can be congenital (e.g. naevi, Mongolian (blue) spots; Figure 14.5) or acquired (post-inflammatory pigmentation). Hypopigmentation (decreases of pigmentation; Figure 14.6) or depigmentation (loss of pigmentation) indicates a congenital (e.g. albinism) or acquired (e.g. vitiligo) disorder in melanin production. In some cases, e.g. tuberous sclerosis, both hyper- and hypopigmented lesions co-exist.

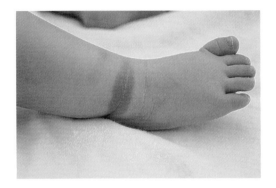

FIGURE 14.5 Mongolian spots.

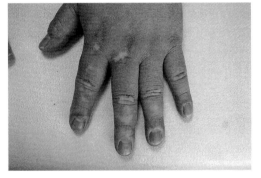

FIGURE 14.6 Hypopigmentation patches.

Possible Diagnoses

Infants	Children
Common	
Carotenaemia	Freckles (ephelides)
Café-au-lait	Lentigines
Mongolian spots	Café-au-lait
Post-inflammatory hyperpigmentation	Post-inflammatory hyperpigmentation (PIH)
Systemic disease, e.g. tuberous sclerosis	Congenital melanocytic naevi (CMN)
Rare	
CMN	Halo naevi
Giant or small hairy naevus	Melanoma
McCune–Albright syndrome	Incontinentia pigmenti
Congenital Addison's disease	Peutz–Jeghers syndrome
Fanconi's syndrome	LEOPARD syndrome
Generalised hereditary lentigines	LAMB syndrome
Androgen excess	Addison's disease/adrenoleukodystrophy)

(Continued)

(Continued)

Infants	Children
	Systemic diseases (e.g. tuberous sclerosis)
	McCune–Albright syndrome
	Haemochromatosis
	Fanconi's syndrome
	Androgen excess
	Drugs (bleomycin, phenytoin, chlorpromazine)
	Acanthosis nigricans
	Morphea (localised scleroderma)
	Pregnancy

Differential Diagnosis at a Glance

	Freckles	Lentigines	Café-au-lait	PIH	CMN
Present at birth	No	Yes	Yes	No	Yes
Sun-exposed area	Yes	No	No	No	No
Previous skin inflammation	No	No	No	Yes	No
Positive family history	Yes	Yes	Yes	No	No
Size >1 cm	No	Yes	Yes	Yes	Yes

Recommended Investigations

No special investigations are usually required in the vast majority of lesions. In some specific cases:

** Biopsy of suspicious lesions (e.g. melanoma) with a few millimetres surrounding of normal skin

Top Tips

- Freckles are dark or brown macules, 2–3 mm in diameter, with poorly defined margins that occur in sun-exposed areas: face, upper back, arms and hands. Lentigines, in contrast to freckles, are larger in size than freckles, unrelated to sun exposure and remain permanently. Both are benign.
- A single café-au-lait spot is a common finding (5%–10%) in Caucasian children. Multiple (more than six) spots suggest neurofibromatosis and are associated with other syndromes such as McCune–Albright syndrome.
- A single small (<1.5 cm) CMN is common and found in 1%–6% of neonates. It is benign and the risk of malignant change in small and medium CMN is less than 1%.
- LAMB syndrome is characterised by facial lentigines in addition to atrial myxoma, mucocutaneous myxoma and blue naevi.
- LEOPARD syndrome consists of lentigines, in association with ECG abnormalities, ocular hypertelorism, pulmonary stenosis, abnormal genitalia, growth retardation and deafness.
- Peutz–Jeghers syndrome consists of hyperpigmented macules, in association with gastrointestinal (GI) polyposis.
- Mastocytosis is a group of disorders that are characterised by an accumulation of mast cells in the skin and other organs. Mastocytoma: a benign cutaneous tumour occurring exclusively in infancy; urticaria pigmentosa: multiple small salmon-coloured or red, cutaneous papules; systemic mastocytosis: mast cell infiltrates in the skin, lymph nodes, liver, spleen, bone and GI tract.

Red Flags

- Carotenaemia – yellow discolouration of the infant skin by the pigment carotene – is often mistaken as jaundice. It occurs in healthy and thriving infants with normal, not jaundiced, sclera.
- Lifetime risk of malignant tumours arising from peripheral nerves in neurofibromatosis is estimated to be 10%–15%. Close observation of individuals with this disease is important.
- Multiple café-au-lait spots are associated with other syndromes (e.g. McCune–Albright syndrome, LEOPARD syndrome, ataxia telangiectasia) which carry a high risk of cancer development.
- Change in the size of CMN occurs normally in proportion to the child's growth and should not be considered as a sign of melanoma. Rapid growth, colour variation and ulceration are red flags.
- Multiple CMN surrounded by satellite naevi and large lesions are considered a risk factor for melanoma and bone and CNS involvement. Excessive exposure to sunlight increases the risk.
- Children with Peutz–Jeghers syndrome are at risk of GI malignancy; a close watch is essential.
- Acanthosis nigricans can suggest insulin resistance and pre-diabetes.

HYPOPIGMENTATION

Possible Diagnoses

Infants	Children
Common	
Naevus depigmentosus	Vitiligo
Partial albinism (piebaldism)	Post-inflammatory hypopigmentation
Naevus anemicus	Pityriasis alba
Menkes' syndrome	Albinism
	Post-varicella depigmentation
Rare	
	Linear lichen sclerosus
	Waardenburg's syndrome
	Chediak-Higashi syndrome
	Ash leaf spots of tuberous sclerosis
	Infectious hypopigmentation (e.g. tinea versicolour)

Differential Diagnosis at a Glance

	Vitiligo	PIH	Pityriasis	Albinism	Post-Varicella Hypopigmentation
Exposed area	No	No	Yes	Yes	No
May present at birth	No	No	No	Yes	No
Sharply demarcated	Yes	No	No	No	No
Inherited	Possible	No	No	Yes	No
Mainly on trunk	No	No	No	No	Yes

Recommended Investigations

No special investigations are usually required in the vast majority of lesions as the diagnosis is mostly clinical. In some specific cases:

**   A skin scrape to differentiate tinea versicolour from hypopigmented spots of pityriasis alba

**   Autoantibody screen may be carried out for vitiligo

***   Wood's light examination to differentiate between depigmented and hypopigmented lesions

***   Cranial MRI or head CT in cases of possible tuberous sclerosis

Top Tips

- Albinism is a hypopigmented disorder involving the skin, hair and iris.
- Vitiligo is a depigmented disorder with an estimated prevalence of 0.5%–1%. It is less frequently associated with autoimmune and endocrine diseases compared to adults. It is, however, associated with a high prevalence of psychological trauma and low self-esteem.

- About one-half of patients with vitiligo have their lesions during childhood. Antibodies to melanocytes are frequently found, suggesting autoimmune cause. A number of autoimmune diseases occur in the patients and their relatives.
- Pityriasis alba is a common condition characterised by ill-defined hypopigmented spots, 1–2 cm in diameter, on the face, arms and neck.

Red Flags

- Be aware that the lack of protective melanin leads children with albinism to high sun sensitivity which results in a high incidence of basal and squamous cell carcinoma. Children with albinism must therefore learn to protect themselves against sun exposure.
- In children with widespread albinism, visual impairment is the rule; the more severe the hypopigmentation, the more severe is the visual acuity.
- Patients with vitiligo lesions have to be told that lesions may progress to become universal.
- Naevus anemicus (an area of localised vasoconstriction) should not be mistaken as ash leaf hypopigmentation: the former is blanchable, while the latter does not disappear on blanching.
- Acanthosis nigricans can suggest insulin resistance and pre-diabetes.

FURTHER READING

Gianfaldonis S, Wollina U, Tcchenev G et al. Vitiligo in children: A review of conventional treatment. *Open Access Maced J Med Sci* 2018;6(1):213–217.

Price HN, Schaffer JV. Congenital melanocytic nevi – When to worry and how to treat: Facts and controversies. *Clin Dermatol* 2010;28(3):293–302.

Russak JE, Dinulos JGH. Pigmented lesions in children. *Semin Plast Surg* 2006;20(3):169–179.

ITCHING (PRURITIS)

Clinical Overview

Pruritis is the most common cutaneous symptom in children characterised by a sensation that provokes a desire to relieve it by scratching. It is either localized, where the diagnosis is easy, or generalised due to systemic disease, where the diagnosis is not obvious and often difficult to establish. In contrast to adults, generalised pruritis due to systemic diseases (e.g. liver, diabetes, renal) is rare in children, with the exception of dry skin, which is very often inherited as an autosomal dominant. The most common two causes of pruritis in children are dry skin and atopic dermatitis (AD). The perianal area (nappy rash, AD, threadworms), vulva (vulvovaginitis) and hair areas (pediculoses, scabies) are the common localised sites of itching.

Possible Diagnoses

Infants	Children
Common	
Atopic dermatitis	Atopic dermatitis
Congenital cholestatic jaundice	Food allergy
Too warm environment	Dry skin (xerosis)
Scabies	Scabies and pediculoses, insects, worms (Figure 14.7)
Dry skin (xerosis)	Urticaria (Figure 14.8)
Rare	
Hyper IgE syndrome	Drugs (e.g. chlorpromazine)
	Cholestasis, hepatitis
	Endocrine (type 1 diabetes)
	Dermatitis herpetiformis
	Psychogenic
	Iron-deficiency anaemia
	Polycythaemia
	Hyper IgE syndrome
	Chronic renal failure
	Lichen planus
	HIV infection
	Pregnancy
	Sea bather's eruption
	Certain malignancy (e.g. Hodgkin's lymphoma)
	Serum sickness

Differential Diagnosis at a Glance

	AD	Food Allergy	Dry Skin	Parasites	Urticaria
Generalised	No	Yes	Yes	No	Yes
Mainly on flexures	Yes	No	No	No	No
Worse at night	Yes	No	Possible	Yes	No
Cause obvious on skin	Yes	No	Yes	Possible	Yes
Positive family history	Yes	Possible	Yes	Possible	No

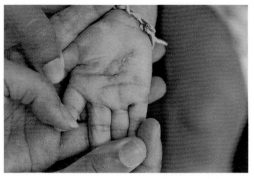
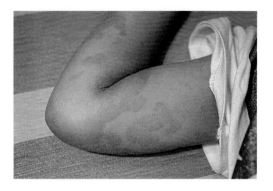

FIGURE 14.7 Itchy skin caused by scabies infestation.   **FIGURE 14.8** Urticaria.

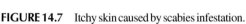

Recommended Investigations

** Fasting blood sugar, urinalysis and hemoglobin A1C to identify diabetes mellitus
** FBC to confirm anaemia or eosinophilia in allergic conditions
** Urea and electrolytes will diagnose chronic renal failure
** LFT: in jaundiced patients
** Thyroid function tests (TFTs) to confirm hypothyroidism or hyperthyroidism
** Scrapings from a burrow to diagnose scabies

Top Tips

- The vast majority of conditions causing pruritus are obvious; the diagnosis is entirely clinical and based on the nature, distribution and duration of the lesions.
- Seborrhoeic dermatitis (SD) is often difficult to differentiate from AD: pruritus is always present in AD, in contrast to SD.
- AD is the most common skin disease in paediatrics (Figure 14.9). It is a chronic, relapsing, highly pruritic condition, affecting 10%–20% of children, commonly associated with elevated IgE levels and *Staphylococcal aureus* colonisation.
- Pruritus is always present in AD; if absent, the diagnosis is incorrect. There is no cure or short cut to the long-term management aimed at relieving the symptoms, including the itching.

Red Flags

- Infants with restlessness, discomfort and excessive crying, particularly at night, may well have pruritic systemic diseases such as non-icteric cholestasis.
- An AD which does not respond to conventional treatment is very often due to *Staphylococcal aureus* or, less commonly, fungal infections. Improvement should occur with antibiotic or anti-fungal treatment even in the absence of clear signs of infection.
- Any skin dermatosis with intense pruritus, particularly when the child is in bed, should alert the physician of the presence of scabies.
- Eczema herpeticum resulting from dissemination of herpes simplex virus in AD can cause kerato-conjunctivitis and multi-organ involvement leading to death. Prompt recognition and anti-viral treatment are essential. Risk factors for this infection include severe AD and marked IgE elevation.

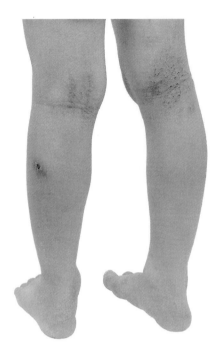

FIGURE 14.9   Atopic dermatitis.

- Generalised pruritis could be the only symptom of obstructive jaundice before the jaundice appears (e.g. primary biliary cirrhosis, drugs), and that of chronic renal failure.
- Any perianal or perineal pruritis at night should alert the clinician to the presence of worms. Inspection of the area by parents while the child is asleep often confirms the diagnosis.
- Children presenting with pruritis of the hair with pyoderma and cervical and occipital lymphadenopathy should be regarded as having pediculosis capitis until proved otherwise. Treatment is urgent.
- Investigation of pruritis is essential for children who are both without physical findings and not responding to a short course of anti-pruritic therapy.

FURTHER READING

Lyons JJ, Milner JD, Stone KD. Atopic dermatitis in children: Clinical features, pathophysiology and treatment. *Immunol Allergy Clin North Am* 2015;35(1):161–183.

MACULES AND PATCHES

Clinical Overview

A macule, known in layman's language as a dot, is a circumscribed, flat area of change in skin colour that is <1 cm in diameter. It can be either hyperpigmented (e.g. freckles) or hypopigmented (vitiligo). Patch is a larger area of change in skin colour that is >1 cm in diameter. The appearance of macules or patches does not commonly remain static, and acute eruptions can change rapidly to become elevated (maculopapular) or blistering (maculovesicular). Therefore, initial rashes which may not be diagnosed on day 1 may be diagnosed on the following day when the rash reaches its ultimate evolution of appearance.

Possible Diagnoses

Infants	Children
Common	
Mongolian spots	Freckles
Cutis marmorata	Bruises
Salmon patch	Viral exanthem
Congenital melanocytic naevus	Drug eruption
Nappy rash	Café-au-lait spots (neurofibromatosis type 1 [NF1])
Rare	
Port-wine stains	Port-wine stains
Tuberous sclerosis (hypopigmented ash leaf)	Cellulitis
	Albinism
	Tuberous sclerosis
	Post-inflammatory hyper- or depigmentation
	Vitiligo
	Intertrigo (inflammatory patch, e.g. in axilla)
	Pityriasis (alba, rubra pilaris)
	Lentigo (benign hyperplasia of melanocytes)
	Tinea versicolour
	Erythema migrans (Lyme disease; Figure 14.10)
	Rheumatic diseases
	Morphea (localised scleroderma)

Differential Diagnosis at a Glance

	Freckles	Bruises	Viral Exanthem	Café-au-lait	Drug Eruption
Fever	No	No	Yes	No	Possible
Blanch on pressure	No	No	Yes	No	Possible
Present at birth	No	No	No	Yes	No
Induced by sunlight	Yes	No	No	No	No
Inherited	Yes	No	No	Possible	No

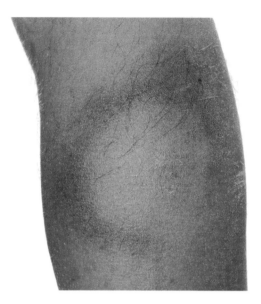

FIGURE 14.10   Erythema migrans.

Recommended Investigations

*** Wood's lamp examination to enhance visualization of hypopigmented lesions
*   Skin scrapings may be required for a suspected case of tinea versicolour
*   Acute and post-convalescent serum samples are occasionally required to confirm rubella
*** Brain imaging to assess for features of Sturge-Weber syndrome or tuberous sclerosis

Top Tips

- Because a specific dermatological diagnosis cannot always be made, classification of a child's skin disease into one of several groups (e.g. as maculopapular, vesico-bullous) is a good start.
- Although blue spots are considered benign, widespread extra-sacral lesions may persist into adulthood. They may co-exist with some inborn errors of metabolism, e.g. gangliosidosis.
- Salmon patch is by far the most common vascular lesion in neonates – a midline or symmetrical pink maculae over both eyelids.
- Single or a couple of café-au-lait lesions, 1–3 cm in diameter occur in about 20% of all healthy children. Café-au-lait spots, the hallmark of NF1, should be six or more café-au-lait spots over 0.5 cm in diameter in pre-pubertal and 1.5 cm in diameter in post-pubertal individuals.
- Café-au-lait spots are one of seven cardinal diagnostic criteria in NF1 that is associated with numerous complications including tumours: neurofibroma, pheochromocytoma and optic glioma.
- Congenital melanocytic naevus (Figure 14.11) occurs in 1%–6% of all neonates; melanomas may rarely develop from these naevi, spontaneous regression may occur.
- Pityriasis versicolour can be hypopigmented (which needs to be differentiated from vitiligo if they appear around the lips) and hyperpigmented.

Red Flags

- Freckles around the mouth should be differentiated from Peutz–Jeghers syndrome. The latter is an autosomal dominant inherited syndrome with hyperpigmented macules on the lip and oral mucosa and is associated with intestinal cancer.

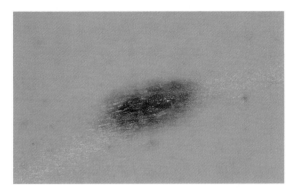

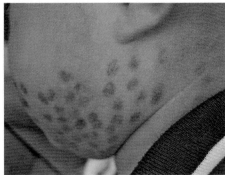

FIGURE 14.11   Congenital melanocytic naevus.   **FIGURE 14.12**   Port-wine stains.

- The oral mucosa hyperpigmented lesions of Peutz–Jeghers syndrome are also found in Addison's disease and McCune–Albright syndrome. Differentiation between these three diseases is essential.
- Port-wine naevus is always present at birth (Figure 14.12). When it is localised to the trigeminal area of the face, the diagnosis is Sturge-Weber syndrome. Be aware of glaucoma and seizure as complications.
- Lesions of pityriasis alba may be mistaken as vitiligo. The borders of the lesions of pityriasis are not sharply demarcated as in vitiligo. Patients and parents of pityriasis can be reassured that complete restoration of normal skin colour will occur.
- Although patches of bruises over the shins are almost universal in toddlers due to frequent falls, bruises on the arm, back, abdomen, thighs and genitalia are suspicious for child abuse.

FURTHER READING

Boyd KP, Korf BR, Theos A. Neurofibromatosis type 1. *J Am Acad Dermatol* 2009;6(1):1–6.

NODULES AND TUMOURS

Clinical Overview

A nodule (lump or bump) is a palpable solid or cystic raised lesion, >1.0 cm in diameter, that extends deeper than a papule: examples are small fibroma, erythema nodosum and skin tumour. Larger nodules >20 mm are classified as tumours, whether benign or malignant. Nodules and tumours are circumscribed, elevated lesions that are larger than papules, which arise from deeper structures, thus displaying elevation as well as depth. Tumours can arise from deeper as well as superficial structures such as dermis or the epidermis.

Possible Diagnoses

Infants	Children
Common	
Warts	Haemangioma (Figure 14.13)
Subcutaneous fat necrosis	Dermoid cyst
Dermoid cyst	Nodulo-cystic acne (Figure 14.14)
Haemangioma	Erythema nodosum
Infantile digital fibroma	Fibroma
Rare	
Mastocytoma	Keloid
Neonatal lupus erythematosus	Discoid lupus erythematosus
Metastatic neuroblastoma	Nasal glioma
Reticulohistiocytosis (Hasimoto-Pritzker disease)	Fibro-sarcoma, basal cell carcinoma
Infantile fibro-sarcoma	Cystic hygroma
	Epidermal naevus
	Mastocytoma
	Subungual/periungual fibroma
	Lipoma
	Juvenile xanthogranuloma
	Hidradenitis
	Rheumatoid nodule
	Malignant melanoma
	Erythema nodosum
	Pyogenic granuloma
	Leishmaniasis, cutaneous
	Xanthoma
	Malignant melanoma
	Sarcoidosis, cutaneous
	Juvenile xanthogranuloma
	Naevus (such as Spitz or sebaceous naevus)

Differential Diagnosis at a Glance

	Fibroma	Dermoid Cyst	Nodulocystic Acne	Erythema Nodosum	Haemangioma
Present in neonate	Possible	Yes	No	No	Yes
Skin coloured	Yes	Yes	No	No	No
Positive comedones	No	No	Yes	No	No
Tenderness	No	No	Possible	Yes	No
Regress	Possible	No	Yes	Yes	Yes

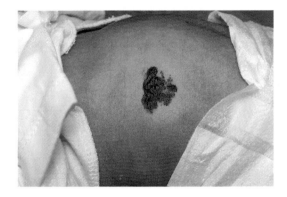

FIGURE 14.13   Haemangioma.

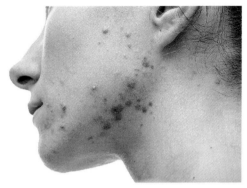

FIGURE 14.14   Nodulocystic acne.

Recommended Investigations

** Urinalysis to detect proteinuria
** FBC: may reveal anaemia in case of chronic inflammatory diseases
** Rheumatoid factor: positive with the presence of rheumatoid nodules
** Kveim test: a useful test in case of sarcoidosis
** Biopsy for obscure nodular lesion

Top Tips

- Haemangiomas are found in about 10% of all children. They are usually not present at birth, appear in the first few weeks of life, enlarge during early infancy and regress aged 4–6 years.
- Syndromes associated with hemagiomas of the face, head or neck include PHACE syndrome, an acronym denoting posterior fossa brain malformation, haemangioma, arterial lesions, cardiac and eye abnormalities.
- Erythema nodosum is an important skin lesion characterised by subcutaneous, tender nodules on the lower legs. The underlying cause may be streptococcal infection, tuberculosis, sarcoidosis or drugs.
- Mastocytoma occurs in infancy as a reddish or orange nodule, rubbery in consistency. A helpful diagnosis clue is Darier's sign: rubbing the lesion releases mast cell mediators, e.g. histamine, resulting in local pruritis, erythema, oedema and blistering.
- Keloid, in contrast to hypertrophic scar, extends its growth beyond the limit of the original scar and does not regress spontaneously. Both result from trauma to the skin, e.g. surgical procedure.

Red Flags

- Although a dermoid cyst is usually benign and most commonly localised on the lateral third of the eyebrow, local growth may cause proptosis, eyelid displacement and erosions on the bone.
- Infantile digital fibroma – a benign, firm, skin-coloured nodule at the lateral surfaces of the distal phalanges – should not be mistaken for a subungual/periungual fibroma found in tuberous sclerosis.
- Any congenital midline lesion, e.g. on the nasal bridge (dermoid cyst, glioma or encephalocele), should be imaged because of the high incidence of intracranial connection. If there

is a sinus opening with intermittent discharge, this is a pathognomonic sign for intracranial connection.

• Although basal cell carcinoma is rare in children, it may result from basal cell naevus, radiotherapy for other malignancies or excessive sun exposure.

• Although paediatric melanoma is rare (1%–4% of all melanomas), its incidence is increasing. The traditional criteria ABCDE (asymmetry, border irregularity, colour changes, diameter >6 mm, evolution) is different in paediatrics: amelanocytic, bleeding, colour uniformity and any size.

• Rhabdomyosarcoma – the most common childhood soft tissue sarcoma – is often mistaken for haemangioma, both clinically and radiologically, due to their vascular pattern. Any firm palpable lesion requires biopsy even if the radiological signs support the diagnosis of haemangioma.

FURTHER READING

Fogelson SK, Dohil MA. Papular and nodular skin lesions in children. *Semin Plast Surg* 2006;20(3):180–191.

PAPULES AND PLAQUES

Clinical Overview

A papule – a little bump or pimple in layman's terms – is a small (<1 cm), solid, circumscribed lesion that is palpable above the skin surface. A plaque is a solid, circumscribed lesion with its surface area greater than the elevation. Plaques vary in size from 1 cm to a huge size covering part of the body. Plaques can arise directly from the skin or through a coalescence of papules. Some eruption has a combination of papules and plaques (papulo-squamous eruption); pityriasis rosea is a typical eruption of this combination.

Possible Diagnoses

Infants	Children
Common	
Erythema toxicum neonatorum	Acne
Milia	AD
Neonatal acne	Warts
AD	Molluscum contagiosum
	Insect bites
Rare	
Histiocytosis syndrome (histiocytosis X)	AD
Mastocytosis	Scabies
	Hand-foot-mouth disease
	Herpes simplex cold sore
	Contact dermatitis
	Papular gloves and socks syndrome
	Discoid lupus erythematosus
	Papular urticaria
	Psoriasis
	Lichen planus
	Histiocytosis syndrome (histiocytosis X)
	Fungal infection
	Keratosis pilaris
	HIV infection

Differential Diagnosis at a Glance

	Acne	AD	Warts	Molluscum	Insect Bite
Severe itching	No	Yes	No	No	Possible
Associated pain	No	No	No	No	Yes
Exposed area	Yes	No	Yes	No	Yes
Adolescence age	Yes	No	No	Yes	No
Umbilicated centre	No	No	No	Yes	No

Recommended Investigations

No special tests are usually required in majority of lesions. Occasional skin lesion may require:

** Scraping of scabies burrow
** Skin biopsy (occasionally may be required)

Top Tips

- Milia – white papules of retention cysts, 1–2 mm in size – are common in neonates (about 50%), seen on the nose and disappear quickly. A pearly papule 1–2 mm on the midline of the palate, Ebstein pearl, is a milium.
- Acne may appear in newborns as self-limited neonatal acne during 0–6 weeks of life, characterised by papulo-vesicular eruption on the face, scalp and neck. Acne also appears in pre-adolescents (7–12 years) and adolescents (12–18 years, affecting about 85% of this age group).
- AD presents during the first 6 months of life as weeping papulo-vesicular eruption on the face and scalp, spreading to the extensor surface of limbs, and to flexural parts.
- Pityriasis rosea is common: self-limited papulo-squamous dermatosis localised mainly on the trunk and often preceded by solitary 'herald sign'. It presents with either papules or plaques.
- Psoriasis is a T-lymphocyte chronic inflammatory disease. About one-third of patients are children. It may present in infancy as a nappy rash. Guttate psoriasis is the most common presentation in older children, characterised by sudden-onset small red or pink papules 1–10 mm in diameter.
- Lichen planus is not that uncommon in children. Lesions are polygonal, flat-topped papules, 2–6 mm in diameter. Diagnosis can often be confirmed by white papules on the buccal mucosa.
- Mastocytosis – accumulation of mast cells in the skin – can present either as disseminated plaques or in solitary, nodular form (mastocytoma).

Red Flags

- Erythema toxicum neonatorum, seen in about half of healthy newborns, is often mistaken as staphylococcal pustules. A well-appearing child and an asymptomatic rash exclude any infection.
- Pre-adolescent acne may precede other signs of puberty maturation. Investigation is unnecessary unless there are signs of androgen excess, polycystic ovarian syndrome or other systemic signs.
- Although hand-foot-mouth disease is usually benign, eruption caused by enterovirus type 71 can spread rapidly causing neurological complications, e.g. encephalitis and spondylitis.
- Scabies is often mistaken as AD or impetigo leading to *Staphylococcus* and *Streptococcus* bacterial infection and subsequently glomerulonephritis and rheumatic fever.
- Histiocytosis (formerly histiocytosis X) can be mistaken as the more common SD if it affects the scalp or AD. The disease has serious complications.

FURTHER READING

Picardo M, Eichenfield LF, Tan J. Acne and rosacea. *Dermatol Ther* 2017;7(Suppl 1):43–52.
Siegfried EC, Herbert AA. Diagnosis of atopic dermatitis: Mimics, overlaps, and complication. *J Clin Med* 2015;4(5):884–917.

PURPURA (PETECHIAE AND ECCHYMOSIS)

Clinical Overview

Purpura indicates extravasation of blood into the skin or mucosal membranes. Lesions are not raised. It may represent a benign condition or a serious underlying disorder. Depending on their size, purpuric lesions are either petechiae (pinpoint haemorrhages <1 cm, usually <2 mm, in diameter) or ecchymoses (>1 cm in diameter). In contrast to exanthem and telangiectasia, purpura does not blanch on pressure. The normal haemostatic mechanisms are complex but primarily are based on vascular response: extravasation is followed by vasoconstriction and retraction of blood vessels to decrease blood flow to the affected area, platelet clot formation and activation of coagulation factors to form fibrin to stabilise the clot. Therefore, purpura is due to vasculopathy, thrombocytopathy, coagulopathy or a combination of these mechanisms. In neonates, petechiae over the presenting part are common, particularly if the delivery was traumatic. In late infancy and toddlers, bruises frequently occur over bony prominences such as shins, knees and forehead.

Possible Diagnoses

Infants	Children
Common	
Infection (intrauterine or acquired)	Henoch–Schönlein purpura (HSP)
Hypoxia (DIC)	Immune thrombocytopenic purpura (ITP)
Drugs	Physical abuse, trauma
Vitamin K deficiency	Infection (e.g. meningococcal septicaemia [MCS])
Congenital thrombocytopenic purpura	Drugs
Rare	
Child abuse	Bone marrow infiltration/failure (e.g. leukaemia)
Thrombocytopenia, absent radius (TAR)	Vascular purpuras (e.g. Von Willebrand's disease)
Kasabach-Merritt syndrome	Hereditary coagulation defects (haemophilia A and B)
(thrombocytopenia with haemangioma)	Ehlers-Danlos syndrome
Wiskott-Aldrich syndrome	Liver disease
Histiocytosis	Malabsorption
Neonatal purpura fulminans	Haemolytic uraemic syndrome
	Scurvy
	Wiskott-Aldrich syndrome
	Post-transfusion purpura

Differential Diagnosis at a Glance

	HSP	ITP	Drugs	MCD	Trauma/ Child Abuse
Petechial	No	Yes	Possible	Yes	No
Low platelets	No	Yes	Possible	Possible	No
Fever	No	No	No	Yes	No
Ill looking	Possible	No	No	Yes	No
Preceded by upper respiratory tract infection	Possible	Yes	No	Possible	No

Recommended Investigations

*** Urine to screen for renal involvement in HSP
*** FBC: for thrombocytopenia, aplastic anaemia, leukocytosis or infection
*** Blood culture, U&E, Ca, blood glucose, FDP for ill children with suspected septicaemia
** Cerebrospinal fluid in cases of meningococcal septicaemia
** LFT and U&E for underlying renal and liver disease
** Coagulation screen: bleeding and clotting time, partial thromboplastin time (PTT) and prothrombin time (PT)
** Fibrin degradation products for DIC
*** Bone marrow examination is occasionally indicated if the cause is not obvious

Top Tips

- In a neonate with petechiae, management starts by taking the mother's previous medical history for presence of ITP, SLE, drugs and infections during pregnancy. In purpura, careful history and thorough examination are more important than extensive tests.
- Baseline tests for most purpuras should include FBC, peripheral blood smear, PT and PTT. Additional tests should be performed when indicated by the history, physical examination and baseline screening tests.
- HSP (or IgA vasculitis, the new term) is the most common vasculitis in children with IgA immune deposits affecting small blood vessels. Renal involvement occurs in 20%–40% of cases, determining long-term prognosis.
- Distribution of the purpura can offer important clues to the diagnosis: in MCS, lesions are often on the neck and chest; in HSP, the lesions are predominately on the shins, feet and buttocks; in ITP, there is bruising and bleeding from the gums and mucous membranes.
- Kasabach-Merritt syndrome is characterised by vascular lesion (haemangioma), thrombocytopenia and chronic consumption coagulopathy. Platelets are consumed and destroyed within the haemangioma.

Red Flags

- Multiple bruises of varying ages on the lower legs of young children should not be mistaken for child abuse. These are common and of no significance. Some petechial lesions seen on the face and neck can follow severe coughing or vomiting. These may be mistaken as septicaemia.
- Infants up to the age of 3–4 months have physiological prolongation of PTT, and abnormal PT and PTT only occur when coagulation factor levels are <40%.
- Although the prognosis of HSP is usually good, hypertension may develop in the recovery period and nephritis may develop months or years after improvement of the HSP findings.
- Although ITP usually has a good prognosis, intracranial haemorrhage occurs in <0.5%, irrespective of the platelet count or treatment given, e.g. corticosteroids or immunoglobulins.
- Of all diseases with purpura and those caused by sepsis, MCS is the most serious and needs urgent management at the emergency room.

- Whenever there are unexplained bruises, non-accidental injury (NAI) should always be suspected. Lesions are suspected when they are found in areas of the body not normally subjected to injury (trunk, buttocks and cheeks). Additional clues for NAI should be sought: inflicted cigarette burns, retinal haemorrhages, intraoral injury and skeletal examination. Radiological skeletal survey may be indicated.
- Any purpura with pallor is likely to be serious: bone marrow disease or haemolytic uraemic syndrome could be the cause. Admit the patient and investigate.

FURTHER READING

Eleftheriou D, Brogan PA. Therapeutic advances in the treatment of vasculitis. *Pediatr Rheumatol Online J* 2016;14:26.

PUSTULES

Clinical Overview

The presence of pustular or vesico-pustular skin lesions on a child's skin is a cause of concern to the family. A pustule is a superficial elevated lesion containing pus. It may primarily result from a bacterial infection, usually staphylococcal, or else when the content of a vesicle or bulla becomes secondarily infected. Pustules are similar to vesicles, but the fluid they contain is purulent exudate. The fluid is the product of accumulation of leukocytes, microorganisms and cellular debris. It may occur either as a primary (e.g. bullous impetigo) or secondary infection of another skin condition (infected AD). When pustules arise at the opening of hair follicles, the condition is termed *folliculitis*. Not all pustules have infectious contents; for example, the contents of transient neonatal pustulosis are sterile without microorganisms if cultured.

Possible Diagnoses

Infants	Children
Common	
Erythema toxicum neonatorum	Infected AD
Staphylococcal infection	Impetigo
Benign neonatal pustulosis	Acne
Bullous impetigo	Varicella (Figure 14.15)
Neonatal acne	Staphylococcal skin infection (e.g. furuncle, carbuncle)
Rare	
Congenital syphilis	Scabies
Congenital varicella	Infected pediculoses
Transient neonatal pustular melanosis	Pyoderma gangrenosum
	Infantile acropustulosis
	Relapse of neonatal herpes simplex virus infection
	Staphylococcal pustulosis

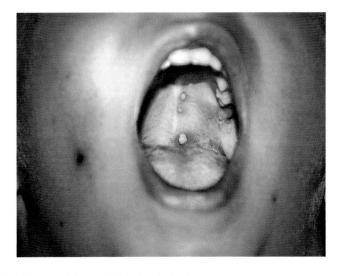

FIGURE 14.15   Vesicles caused by varicella virus infection.

Differential Diagnosis at a Glance

	Infected AD	Impetigo	Acne	Varicella	Staphylococcal Skin Infection
Presence of comedones	No	No	Yes	No	No
Mucosal involvement	No	No	No	Yes	No
Fever	Possible	No	No	Yes	Possible
Severe pruritis	Yes	Possible	Possible	Yes	Possible
Perioral involvement	No	Yes	No	No	No

Recommended Investigations

No special investigations are usually required in the vast majority of lesions as the diagnosis is mostly clinical. In some specific cases:

** Swab from any pus or open infected lesion to confirm the organism
** Polymerase chain reaction analysis of pustular fluid for herpes simplex virus or varicella zoster virus

Top Tips

- Not all pustules indicate infection as some fluids inside are sterile when cultured, e.g. benign neonatal pustulosis and transient neonatal pustular melanosis. Both are self-limited dermatosis of unknown aetiology and require no treatment.
- Important bacterial causes of pustules include bullous impetigo, folliculitis and ecthyma (deeper infection than impetigo). Direct examination of the lesion scraping and staining by Gram can identify the presence of Gram-positive bacteria such as streptococci and staphylococci.
- Papules and pustules around the mouth (impetigo) are often due to staphylococcal or streptococcal infection and should be treated with an antibiotic and not with topical steroid.

Red Flags

- Erythema toxicum neonatorum may be predominately pustular; therefore, they must be differentiated from similar appearing lesions of staphylococcal infection.
- It is important to differentiate neonatal varicella (NV) from congenital varicella syndrome (CVS). CVS occurs when pregnant women contract varicella at 6–20 weeks of gestation, causing in about 25% of neonates varicella embryopathy (such as limb interruption, eye involvement, cicatricial scarring). NV occurs if the fetus is born within a week of maternal varicella, resulting in a severe form of varicella because of the lack of transplacental antibody to the virus.
- Early diagnosis of congenital syphilis may be difficult as babies may present with subtle and non-specific symptoms including rhinitis, generalised erythematous macules and papulo-pustular skin rash on the palms and soles. An X-ray of the long bones showing periostitis is a very important clue.
- Herpes simplex virus infection or zoster in an immunocompromised child indicates serious infection; urgent management and appropriate treatment are required.
- Clinicians should keep scabies in mind in the differential diagnosis in a child who presents with purpuric vesicular or pustular skin infection. The infection may affect newborns with associated findings of irritability, poor feeding and weight loss.

FURTHER READING

Reginatto FP, Villa DD, Cestari TF. Benign skin disease with pustules in the newborn. *An Bras Dermatol* 2016;91(2):124–134.

SWEATING, EXCESSIVE (HYPERHIDROSIS)

Clinical Overview

Physiological sweating is a vital process for hypothalamic-controlled thermoregulation; there is also emotional sweating regulated by the limbic system. The human body has about 4 million sweat glands; 75% are eccrine. Eccrine sweat glands, found all over the skin surface, cool the body by evaporation of sweat. Apocrine sweat glands become active during puberty and are mainly present in the axillae, anogenital skin and mammary areas and produce viscous fluid to give the body a distinctive odour. Excessive perspiration (hyperhidrosis) is due to overactive sweat glands as a result of dysregulation of the neural sympathetic control of the eccrine sweat glands. It can be generalised or localised to certain parts of the body such as palms, axillae or soles. It can also be primary, usually idiopathic, or secondary caused by an underlying condition (e.g. hyperthyroidism). Excessive sweating is a common problem and can be distressing; leading to embarrassment and avoidance of social contact.

Possible Diagnoses

Infants	Children
Common	
Warm environment	Fever (phase of defervescence)
Infection	Emotional/anxiety
Drugs (antipyretics)	Drugs (e.g. antipyretics, opioids, fluoxetine)
Warm dressed	Idiopathic
Excessive crying	Obesity
Rare	
Heart failure	Endocrine (e.g. hyperthyroidism, pheochromocytoma)
	Rickets
	Spinal injury
	Heart failure
	Hypoglycaemia
	Familial dysautonomia
	Malignancy (e.g. lymphoma)
	Tuberculosis
	Withdrawal from narcotics, opiates
	Carcinoid syndrome
	Chiari malformation with syringohydromyelia
	Chédiak-Higashi syndrome

Differential Diagnosis at a Glance

	Fever	Emotion/Anxiety	Drugs	Idiopathic	Obesity
Generalised	Yes	No	Yes	Yes	No
Profuse	Yes	Possible	Possible	Yes	Possible
Ill looking	Yes	No	Possible	No	No
Associated pallor	No	Possible	No	No	No
Related to movement	No	No	No	No	Yes

Recommended Investigations

The vast majority of cases with hyperhidrosis do not require any investigation as the cause is obvious.

*** Blood for TFTs, blood glucose to confirm, e.g. hyperthyroidism or hypoglycaemia
*** Hyperhidrosis severity scale: to monitor progress after initiating treatment
*** Brain and cervical MRI in cases of suspected Chiari malformation

Top Tips

- Palmar hyperhidrosis has a prevalence of up to 3% of the population. In situations with fever, anxiety and stress there will be worsening symptoms.
- In children with acute hyperhidrosis, febrile illness is by far the most common cause.
- In cases of generalised sweating, every effort should be made to find an underlying systemic cause (e.g. hyperthyroidism, or hypoglycaemia) and treat it.
- In excessive sweating of the palms and soles, aluminum hydrochloride as a 20% solution is often helpful.
- The low social esteem and social isolation experienced by some patients with hyperhidrosis may be compounded by the malodorous (bromhidrosis) and fetid odour caused by decomposition of the sweat by bacteria and yeasts.

Red Flags

- Be aware that in severe cases of sweating, the skin, especially on the feet, may be macerated, fissured and scaling. This can be mistakenly diagnosed as a primary infection such as fungal infection rather than sweating as the primary cause. Increased hydration may contribute to pyogenic infection and contact dermatitis.
- Episodic sweating, particularly if associated with abdominal symptoms (diarrhoea, vomiting or pain), could have carcinoid syndrome or pheochromocytoma as an underlying cause.
- Sweating, with mild or without obvious fever, can be due to tuberculosis, brucellosis or lymphoma.
- Urgent attention should be given to sweating occurring in sleep or associated with weight loss.

FURTHER READING

Romero FR, Haddad GR, Miot HA et al. Palmar hyperhidrosis: Clinical, pathophysiological, diagnostic and therapeutic aspects. *An Bras Dermatol* 2016;91(6):716–725.

TELANGIECTASIA

Clinical Overview

Telangiectasia indicates permanently dilated superficial blood vessels in the skin or mucous membranes. One or two telangiectases on the face (occasionally on the dorsa of the hands) are common and trivial in children, and highly characteristic in the vascular centre, from which radiates fine vessels that give the appearance of a spider web. Unlike petechiae, which have a similar appearance, they blanch with pressure and refill immediately after the pressure is released. Other lesions may suggest serious systemic disease such as ataxia telangiectasia (progressive cerebellar ataxia, sinopulmonary infection and immunodeficiency) and hereditary haemorrhagic telangiectasia (Osler-Weber-Rendu disease), which is autosomal dominant, characterised by arteriovenous malformation on the skin, mucous membranes and internal organs such as brain, liver and lungs.

Possible Diagnoses

Infants	Children
Common	
	Spider angioma (common telangiectasia)
	Oestrogen treatment/pregnancy
	Liver disease
	Connective tissue diseases
	Hereditary haemorrhagic telangiectasia (HHT)
Rare	
Bloom syndrome	Ataxia telangiectasia
Telangiectatic haemangioma (reticular infantile haemangioma)	Hereditary benign telangiectasia
	Topical steroid treatment
Cutis marmorata telangiectasia	Generalised essential telangiectasia
	CREST syndrome
	Congenital cutis marmorata telangiectasia (CCMT)
	Idiopathic telangiectasia
	Unilateral nevoid telangiectasia
	Chronic sun exposure

Differential Diagnosis at a Glance

	Spider Angioma	Oestrogen Treatment	Liver Disease	Connective Tissue Diseases	HHT
Effect of oestrogen	Yes	Yes	Yes	No	No
Associated with haemorrhage	No	No	Yes	No	Yes
Inherited	No	No	Possible	Possible	Yes
Visceral involvement	No	No	Yes	Possible	Yes
Benign	Yes	Yes	No	No	No

Recommended Investigations

*** LFT to exclude liver disease

** Urinalysis to exclude renal disease in collagen diseases (e.g. SLE)

*** Immunoglobulin for telangiectasia is associated with immunoglobulin deficiency

** Pregnancy test may be needed for widespread telangiectasia and in case of spider angiomas

** Anti-nuclear antibodies (ANAs), SLE double-strand test to exclude SLE for connective diseases

** X-rays of legs may detect calcinosis in CREST (calcinosis, Raynaud's phenomenon, oesophageal dysmotility, sclerodactyly and telangiectasia) syndrome

** Chest X-ray and liver ultrasound in cases of suspected HHT

Top Tips

- Spider angiomas (nevus araneus) are a common condition, occurring in up to 15% of pre-school-aged children and 45% of school-aged children, usually on the cheeks and dorsa of the hands. They often disappear in children and tend to persist in adults.
- Some telangiectasias are not obvious and need to be searched for, e.g. in the bulbar conjunctive in ataxia telangiectasia and on the tongue and mucous membranes in HHT.
- The majority of cases with cutis marmorata are trivial and occur commonly in neonates and infants. More pronounced and persistent lesions during exercise, crying and changes of environmental temperature could well be due to CCMT. This is also benign.
- Telangiectasia is part of CREST syndrome. Two or more of the features of calcinosis, Raynaud's phenomenon, oesophageal dysmotility, sclerodactyly and telangiectasia establish the diagnosis.
- Ataxia telangiectasia manifests soon after children begin to walk with progressive cerebellar ataxia, sinopulmonary symptoms and immunodeficiency. Children are wheelchair bound usually aged 10–12 years. Telangiectasia usually appears aged 3–6 years.
- Bloom syndrome, inherited as an autosomal recessive, mapped to chromosome 15, manifests in infancy as facial erythema and telangiectasia in a butterfly distribution, similar to SLE, after sun exposure.

Red Flags

- The commonly appearing facial telangiectasia should not be linked to any disease, e.g. liver disease, unless they are associated with other symptoms suggestive of an underlying disease.
- Although Raynaud's phenomenon is often benign and due to reactive peripheral vasoconstriction, some children do develop later connective tissue disease, particularly progressive systemic sclerosis and CREST syndrome. Screening for auto-antibodies is useful.
- Children with HHT experience recurrent epistaxis and other haemorrhages (GI, mouth, and lungs) before the typical appearance of telangiectasia, which may develop later. Around 15%–20% of patients present with stroke.
- Iron treatment in HHT may precipitate epistaxis within hours. Reduced strength of the iron tablets may not cause this phenomenon.

FURTHER READING

Shovlin CL, Gilson C, Busbridge M et al. Can Iron treatments aggravate epistaxis in some patients with hereditary haemorrhagic telangiectasia? *Laryngoscope* 2016;126(11):2468–2474.

15 HAIR AND NAILS

ALOPECIA (HAIR LOSS)

Clinical Overview

Hair, derived from the epidermis, develops around the third to fourth months of fetal life. At birth, the number of hair follicles on the scalp (about a million) and on other parts of the body (about 4 million) stabilises and no more follicles are developed. The hair cycle consists of a growing phase of hair (anagen), which lasts about 2–6 years and constitutes about 90% of the total hair, and a resting phase (telogen), which lasts about 3 months. Normally, 30–150 hairs are shed daily from our scalp but hair re-grows automatically so that the total number of hairs remains constant. Alopecia may occur in patches (alopecia areata), on the entire scalp (totalis) or over the entire body (universalis). Alopecia areata is the most common type of alopecia, affecting 1%–2% of the world's population. It is a polygenic autoimmune disease that may be associated with other autoimmune disorders, e.g. thyroid. The prognosis is good as hair follicle bulbs are not destroyed. Some 80%–90% will experience re-growth of their hair within a year. Alopecia may also be scarring (hair follicle is irreversibly destroyed) or non-scarring which has the potential for hair re-growth.

Possible Diagnoses

Infants	Children
Common	
Normal (after lanugo hair shedding)	Alopecia areata (also totalis, universalis)
Pressure alopecia	Tinea capitis (TC)
Seborrhoeic dermatitis	Nutritional (e.g. iron, zinc deficiency)
Hidrotic ectodermal dysplasia	Drugs (e.g. cytotoxic, anticoagulants, anticonvulsants)
Congenital alopecia (autosomal recessive)	Trauma (traction alopecia, compulsive pulling)
Rare	
Syndrome (e.g. Menkes' kinky hair)	Child abuse
Child abuse	Cicatricial alopecia (e.g. lichen planus)
Hereditary vitamin D resistant rickets (HVDRR)	HVDRR
Genetic alopecia	Infection (e.g. typhoid fever, syphilis)
	Short anagen syndrome
	Endocrine (e.g. hypothyroidism, hypopituitarism)
	Genetic alopecia (autosomal recessive)
	Syndromes (e.g. Hallermann-Streiff)
	Metabolic (e.g. homocystinuria)
	Biotinidase deficiency
	Obsessive-compulsive disorder

Differential Diagnosis at a Glance

	Alopecia Areata	Tinea Capitis	Nutritional	Drugs	Trauma
Infancy	No	Possible	Possible	Possible	Possible
Patchy	Yes	Yes	Possible	Possible	Yes
Normal scalp	Yes	No	Possible	Yes	Yes
Pruritis	No	Yes	Possible	No	No
Diagnosis by Wood's light	No	Yes	No	No	No

Recommended Investigations

*** Wood's light confirms tinea infection
*** Thyroid function tests, zinc, iron, total protein and fractions for nutritional causes
*** Autoimmune screen (e.g. anti-nuclear antibodies) for cases of alopecia areata
**   Investigations to exclude possible metabolic causes (e.g. homocystinuria, biotinidase deficiency)

Top Tips

- Patchy alopecia on the occipital or temporal area in a baby is common and is usually due to preferential sleeping on that area. Sweating causes rubbing and worsens the condition.
- When examining a child with alopecia, find out whether it is diffuse or patchy, inflammatory or non-inflammatory, scarring or non-scarring. This will help with the differential diagnosis.
- The diagnostic sign for alopecia areata is 'exclamation mark' hairs, which are 1–2 mm in length, tapered at the attached end and seen at the periphery of new bald patches.
- Nutritional causes of alopecia in developing countries are common, e.g. marasmus (protein-calorie deficiency) or kwashiorkor (protein deficiency).
- Traction alopecia (trauma to hair follicle resulting from traction by tight headbands, ponytails, rollers or curlers) is more common in girls of African descent.
- Trichotillomania is a behavioural disorder characterised by patients recurrently pulling their own hair; it may be part of an obsessive-compulsive disorder (OCD). It is more common in females and in adolescents.
- Telogen effluvium (diffuse form of hair loss) is an increased loss of hair than in normal hair shedding. It may occur following stress or medications (e.g. childbirth, febrile illness, surgery, severe weight loss, discontinuation of high dose of steroids). Hair will re-grow in about 6 months.

Red Flags

- Alopecia areata may affect eyebrows and eyelashes only.
- Be aware that alopecia may be caused by child abuse. The hairs are typically broken at various lengths. Examine the skin carefully for other signs of abuse such as bruises.
- Trichotillomania and TC may be mistaken for alopecia areata. Wood's light is diagnostic for TC.

- For extensive alopecia areata with loss of eyebrows and lashes occurring in early childhood, the prognosis is bad. In the absence of these risk factors, it may take 1 year for the hair to re-grow.
- Any child with alopecia areata should be examined and investigated for other autoimmune disorders such as vitiligo, coeliac disease, diabetes or Addison's disease. Good history is essential.
- Trauma caused by traction of hair follicles (from tight braids or ponytails) is common in girls of school age. They should be encouraged to avoid devices that cause trauma to hair.
- In trichotillomania (compulsive pulling), there is an impulse to pull at the hair. Many children suffer from emotional stress and OCD, often requiring a psychiatric consultation.
- As 30% of patients with trichotillomania have the habit of swallowing the hair, they may present with serious gastrointestinal complaints as the first manifestation of the disease.

FURTHER READING

Pratt CH, King LE, Messenger AG et al. Alopecia areata. *Nat Rev Dis Primers* 2017;3:17011.

BODY HAIR, EXCESSIVE

Clinical Overview

Vellus hair is fine, soft and non-pigmented, and covers most of the body before puberty. Terminal hair, in contrast, is coarse, curly and pigmented. Pubertal androgens promote the conversion from vellus to terminal hair. Hair growth in excess of what is expected for age, sex and ethnicity is termed *hirsutism* or *hypertrichosis*. While hypertrichosis indicates non-androgenic excessive vellus hair growth in areas not usually hairy, hirsutism is an androgen-dependent male pattern of terminal hair growth in women. It may be localised or generalised, transient or permanent. The most common cause of hypertrichosis or hirsutism is racial or familial, which is frequent in people from the Mediterranean area and the Indian subcontinent. It can be idiopathic or drug induced. In this country, the most common cause of hirsutism is polycystic ovary syndrome (PCOS). Important endocrine causes of hirsutism are congenital adrenal hyperplasia (CAH) and Cushing's syndrome.

Possible Diagnoses

Infants	Children
Common	
Lanugo hair (racial)	Racial and familial hypertrichosis or hirsutism
Drugs	Drugs (e.g. steroids, phenytoin, cyclosporine, Minoxidil)
Endocrine (e.g. CAH)	Endocrine causes (e.g. Cushing's syndrome, CAH, adrenal tumour)
Congenital pigmented naevus	PCOS
Congenital melanocyte naevus	Malnutrition, including anorexia nervosa
Rare	
Congenital hypertrichosis	Hyperprolactinaemia
Ambras' syndrome	Pituitary adenoma
Cornelia de Lange syndrome	Cornelia de Lange syndrome
Fetal hydantoin syndrome	Porphyria cutanea tarda
Localised	Sertoli-Leydig cell tumour
	Granulosa-thecal cell tumour
	Congenital terminal hypertrichosis with gingival hyperplasia
	Idiopathic hirsutism
	Paraneoplastic syndrome

Differential Diagnosis at a Glance

	Racial/Familial	Drugs	Endocrine	PCOS	Malnutrition
Positive family history					
Otherwise healthy	Yes	No	No	No	No
Infancy	Yes	Possible	Possible	No	Possible
Recent onset	No	Possible	Possible	No	No
Associated obesity	No	Possible	Possible	Yes	No

Recommended Investigations

*** Urine for porphyria: 24-hour urine collection for cortisol levels in CAH

*** Urea and electrolytes: for salt-losing CAH

*** Serum testosterone, dehydroepiandrosterone sulfate (DHEAS), luteinising hormone, follicle-stimulating hormone: raised in PCOS and tumour
*** Serum 17-hydroxyprogesterone, DHEAS will confirm CAH
*** Serum prolactin to diagnose hyperprolactinaemia
*** Thyroid function tests
*** Ultrasound scan for PCOS and CAH

Top Tips

- Excessive hair growth is mostly racial and familial, so investigation is often not required.
- Although the term *hirsutism* is mostly used in women, remember that hirsutism in pre-pubertal children occurs equally in both sexes. It is an important sign of precocious puberty.
- The benign form of hirsutism is characterised by its pubertal onset and slow progression over many years. PCOS is an example of this and affects 5%–10% of women of reproductive age.
- PCOS usually manifests at puberty with menstrual disturbances, hirsutism, obesity with insulin resistance and evidence of androgen excess (clinically and/or biochemically). PCOS can be associated with the use of certain medications, such as valproic acid.
- Hirsutism, congenital or acquired, is caused by excessive androgen. Patients often have deepening of the voice, acne, irregular menstruation and a masculine body.
- Ultrasonography has an important role to play in this condition, e.g. determining uterus and ovaries in masculine signs of CAH, identification of multicystic ovaries (pearl necklace) in PCOS and detecting ovarian and adrenal tumours.
- Paraneoplastic syndrome is a rare disorder of a wide variety of clinical pictures (e.g. myasthenic syndrome with lung cancer) that occur at sites distant from the tumour.

Red Flags

- Any acute and/or severe hirsutism requires investigation to exclude serious underlying causes such as a tumour of the ovary or adrenal cortex.
- Be aware that, while high levels of testosterone with normal DHEAS indicate that the ovaries are producing the androgens, high levels of testosterone with high DHEAS indicate that the adrenal glands are producing the androgen.
- Hypertrichosis must be distinguished from hirsutism causing virilisation; the latter is associated with acne, increased muscle bulk, deepening of the voice and clitoromegaly.
- In CAH, steroidogenesis takes place *in utero*, so signs of masculinisation (enlarged and fused clitoris, resembling a penis and labial fusion) are present at birth. A mistaken diagnosis of cryptorchidism and hypospadias is often made.
- As patients with PCOS typically have metabolic syndrome, blood pressure and testing for diabetes should not be missed.
- Be aware that female neonates exposed to high levels of androgen *in utero* are at increased risk of developing PCOS in adolescence.

FURTHER READING

Mihaildis J, Demesropian R, Taxel P et al. Endocrine evaluation of hirsutism. *Int J Women Dermatol* 2017;3(1 Suppl):S6–S10.

ITCHY SCALP

Clinical Overview

Examination of the scalp is an important part of the skin examination. Itchy scalp is a common and distressing complaint in paediatrics that can be diagnostically and therapeutically challenging. Itchy scalp is caused by a variety of conditions including systemic (e.g. cholestatic liver disease, renal failure and diabetes), inflammatory (e.g. seborrhoeic and atopic dermatitis, psoriasis, xerosis and lichen planus), infectious (e.g. folliculitis, pediculosis, scabies and insect bites), neoplastic (e.g. naevi and melanoma), autoimmune disease related (e.g. dermatitis herpetiformis) and psychogenic. Of the three types of lice, pediculus humanus capitis, corporis and pubis, pediculosis capitis is the most common and important type. The diagnosis is easy in the vast majority of cases and should be made by thorough examination of the scalp before considering any treatment.

Possible Diagnoses

Infants	Children
Common	
Excessive wrapping	Pediculosis capitis
Scabies	Scabies
Pediculosis capitis	Atopic dermatitis
Cholestasis	Dry skin (xerosis)
Atopic dermatitis	Tinea capitis
Rare	
Poor hygiene including neglect	Poor hygiene
Impetigo	Contact dermatitis
Acute viral infection (e.g. varicella)	Inflammatory (e.g. psoriasis, acne vulgaris)
Drugs (e.g. iron, zinc)	Infection (e.g. impetigo, folliculitis, varicella)
	Discoid lupus
	Lichen simplex (neurogenic excoriation)
	Papular urticaria (insect bites)
	Systemic (e.g. obstructive jaundice, diabetes)
	Drugs (e.g. iron and zinc preparations, opioids)
	Autoimmune disease (e.g. dermatitis herpetiformis)

Differential Diagnosis at a Glance

	Pediculosis	Scabies	Atopic Dermatitis	Xerosis	Tinea Capitis
Positive family history	Possible	Possible	Yes	Yes	No
Skin lesions elsewhere	No	Possible	Yes	Possible	No
Normal hair	Yes	Yes	Yes	Yes	No
Pustules	Possible	Possible	Possible	No	Possible
Dermoscopy diagnostic	Yes	Yes	Possible	No	Yes

Recommended Investigations

** Wood's light of the hair and scalp
** Dermoscopic identification of mites from their burrows in scabies, naevi
** Gram stain and culture from the follicular orifice to identify the bacteria in folliculitis

Top Tips

- In infants, warm wrapping and warm ambient temperature are common causes of restlessness, sweating and scalp pruritis.
- Remember that poor hygiene is often the underlying cause of scalp itching, such as pediculosis. Examination of the child may confirm other areas of his or her body with poor hygiene.
- Bullae, pustules and dermatitis of the skin and scalp dominate in infants with scabies. In older children, small papules and vesicles localised in the interdigital space and wrist flexors are seen.
- Wood's lamp is a useful tool to have: blue-green fluorescence is detectable in the hair shaft infected by fungal infection. *Tinea versicolor* has golden fluorescence. A dark room is needed.
- As lice and ova (nits) are often hard to see in fair hair, the best way to identify lice is to comb the hair properly with a louse comb, preferably from the hairs behind the ears and back of the neck.
- A common cause of scalp pruritis is contact dermatitis due to the use of soaps, shampoo and other hair products, particularly those that contain alcohol.
- Scalp naevi often cause anxiety for professionals and parents. Dermoscopy is a non-invasive tool in the evaluation of these naevi including melanoma.
- In children with impaired immunity (e.g. HIV) or receiving immunosuppressive drugs (e.g. steroids), widespread and serious scabies rash with thick scaling may occur (Norwegian scabies). The mites are able to multiply into thousands. The nails become thickened and dystrophic.

Red Flags

- Although pruritic patchy alopecia is often caused by alopecia areata or tinea capitis, discoid lupus erythematosus and secondary syphilis should be considered in the differential diagnosis.
- Fever, regional lymphadenopathy and widespread pustules caused by bacterial infection often complicate pediculosis, tinea capitis and scalp dermatitis. It is essential to search for the cause of this inflammatory response.
- Remember that some drugs (e.g. iron, zinc and opioids) can directly cause itching; other drugs (e.g. chlorpromazine) may indirectly cause itching by causing obstructive jaundice.
- Melanoma of the scalp is associated with worse prognosis compared to melanomas located elsewhere on the body mainly because of the invisibility of these lesions inside the scalp.

FURTHER READING

Bin Saif GA, Ericson M, Yosipovitch G. The itchy scalp – Searching for an explanation. *Exp Dermatol* 2011;20(12):959–968.
Toheung WJ, Bellet JS, Prose NS et al. Clinical and dermoscopic features of 88 scalp nevi in 30 children. *Br J Dermatol* 2011;165(1):137–143.

NAIL ABNORMALITIES

Clinical Overview

Abnormal nails may occur as a result of generalised skin disease, skin disease confined to the nails, systemic disease, fungal or bacterial infection or tumour. It is important to distinguish between absent or small nails (anonychia) occurring in epidermolysis bullosa, acrodermatitis enteropathica, incontinentia pigmenti or nail-patella syndrome; abnormalities of the nail shape (e.g. koilonychia or clubbing); abnormalities of the nail surface; abnormalities of the nail colour (leukonychia, melanonychia or yellow); and abnormalities of the nail attachment such as onycholysis. Finger clubbing is an important sign for paediatricians and seen in patients with cyanotic congenital heart, pulmonary (e.g. cystic fibrosis) and inflammatory bowel diseases. Splinter haemorrhage is an important clue to subacute bacterial endocarditis.

Possible Diagnoses

Infants	Children
Common	
Koilonychia	Clubbing
Paronychial inflammation	Koilonychia
Small or absent nails	Paronychial inflammation
Trauma	Onycholysis (separation of nail plate from the distal nail bed)
Atopic dermatitis	Onychomycosis (fungal infection)
Rare	
Effect of drugs	Effect of drugs (e.g. chloroquine, bleomycin, vincristine)
Pachyonychia congenita	Psoriatic nails
Nail-patella syndrome	Small or absent nails
	Ingrown nails
	Tumour (e.g. periungual fibroma, subungual melanoma)
	Nail-patella syndrome
	Yellow nail syndrome
	Longitudinal or transverse ridges
	Beau's lines (caused by, e.g. arsenic poisoning)

Differential Diagnosis at a Glance

	Clubbing	Koilonychia	Paronychial Inflammation	Onycholysis	Onychomycosis
May be normal	Yes	Yes	No	No	No
Inherited	Possible	No	No	No	No
Abnormal nail shape	Yes	Yes	Possible	No	Possible
Part of systemic disease	Yes	Yes	No	Yes	No
May be idiopathic	Yes	Yes	No	Possible	No

Recommended Investigations

*** FBC and serum ferritin in spoon-shaped nails to exclude anaemia

**   Throat swab for culture and ASO titre in cases of acute psoriasis (guttate form)

**   Wood's light and microscopy of culture in fungal infection

Top Tips

- Koilonychia (spoon-shaped nails) can be normal during the first 2 years of life and corrects itself later on. An important cause is iron-deficiency anaemia (Plummer-Vinson syndrome).
- Pachyonychia congenita is an autosomal dominant trait associated with hypertrophic nail dystrophy (pachyonychia); it often leads to paronychia, nail loss and keratoderma.
- Small or absent nails may occur in association with nail-patella syndrome, in which the nail size is reduced by 30%–50%. This is an autosomal dominant disease with small and unstable patella.
- Paronychial inflammation may occur after prolonged immersion with water, which may occur with prolonged thumb or finger sucking.
- Nail involvement is a valuable diagnostic sign in psoriasis: pitting of the nail plate, onycholysis and yellow-brown subungual discolouration of the nails.
- Children and adolescents with sub- or periungual fibromas should be examined for additional signs of tuberous sclerosis.

Red Flags

- In paediatrics, nail clubbing is the most important of all nail abnormalities. It is often seen in children with cystic fibrosis, inflammatory bowel diseases, cyanotic congenital heart diseases or bronchiectasis, as well as in healthy people (idiopathic or inherited).
- Nail clubbing may be an early sign of AIDS.
- Remember that the nail plate is relatively pliable and thin during the first 1–2 years of life; thus, spoon-shaped nails (koilonychia) at this age can be normal. Do not mistake them as pathological.
- Both flattening and concavity (koilonychia) and white opacity of the nails (leukonychia) may harbour an underlying disease such as anaemia.
- Onycholysis is often due to trauma or psoriasis. Thyroid disease should also be considered.
- Although subungual splinter haemorrhage (red-brown longitudinal lines resulting from capillary leakage) may occur as a result of trauma or psoriasis, they are a very important clue for subacute bacterial endocarditis. The presence of cardiac murmur and fever clinches the diagnosis.

FURTHER READING

Singal A, Arora R. Nail as a window of systemic diseases. *Indian Dermatol Online J* 2015;6(2):67–74.

16 BONES AND JOINTS

ARTHRALGIA (PAINFUL JOINT)

Clinical Overview

Painful joint (arthralgia) is one of the most common complaints in children, indicating joint pain not accompanied by obvious clinical signs of arthritis. It may be generalised, involving multiple joints, mostly caused by a viral infection, benign growing pain, joint hypermobility or minor trauma. However, arthralgia may be a warning sign of serious underlying diseases, including juvenile idiopathic arthritis (JIA) or haematological malignancies. The best approach to a child with arthralgia and normal examination is to perform careful initial evaluation and inflammatory tests (such as white blood cell [WBC] count, C-reactive protein [CRP]), followed by periodic monitoring for changing in symptoms or physical findings. Steroid treatment should not be used before final diagnosis is established and a malignancy excluded. Parents are usually worried that a rapid diagnosis often cannot be made and that clinicians are not telling them what is wrong with their child; parental concern should be alleviated by informing them there is a programme in place to monitor their child's symptoms.

Possible Diagnoses

Infants	Children
Common	
Acute viral infection	Acute viral infection
Trauma	Trauma
Sickle-cell anaemia (SCA)	Referred pain (knee arthralgia referred from hip)
Child abuse	Pre-arthritic (e.g. JIA)
Malignancy (e.g. leukaemia)	Malignancy (e.g. leukaemia)
Rare	
	SCA
	Vasculitis (e.g. Henoch–Schönlein purpura)
	Child abuse
	Avascular necrosis (e.g. slipped capital femoral epiphysis)
	Brucellosis
	Fabry's disease
	Inflammatory bowel disease (Crohn's disease, colitis)
	Rheumatic fever
	Sarcoidosis
	Drugs (e.g. carbimazole)
	Psychogenic
	Trichinosis
	Hypermobility of connective tissue
	Immunodeficiency (e.g. IgA deficiency)
	Wegener's granulomatosis

Differential Diagnosis at a Glance

	Viral Infection	Trauma	Referred Pain	Pre-arthritic	Malignancy
Mono-arthritis	No	Yes	Yes	No	Possible
Associated fever	Yes	No	Possible	Possible	Possible
Severe persistent pain	No	Possible	No	Possible	Yes
Abnormal full blood count (FBC), high CRP	No	No	Possible	Yes	Yes
Diagnosis by imaging	No	Possible	Possible	Possible	Possible

Recommended Investigations

** FBC with CRP: for bacterial diseases; leucopenia in systemic lupus erythematosus (SLE); blood smear for leukaemia

** CPK: elevated in dermatomyositis

*** Haemoglobin (Hb)-electrophoresis and peripheral film for SCA

** Kveim test for suspected cases of sarcoidosis

*** X-ray: diagnostic for avascular necrosis and excluding avascular necrosis

** Bone scan is sometimes required, e.g. suspected bone tumour

Top Tips

- Every attempt should be made to ensure that there are no signs of arthritis (red, hot and swollen joint) and to localise the arthralgia. Once a joint is found responsible, diagnosis becomes easy.
- Arthralgia of the hip includes transient synovitis, Perthes' disease or slipped capital femoral epiphysis. The latter typically affects obese, short children or those with a rapid growth spurt.
- Painful knee may be caused by traumatic synovitis, haemarthrosis, chondromalacia patella, patellar subluxation or dislocation, synovial plicae, osteochondritis dissecans or tumour.
- Although children with avascular necrosis of the tibia (Osgood-Schlatter syndrome) usually present with pain around the anterior knee, examination often reveals swelling, tenderness and prominence of the tibia tubercle. Healing is usually slow, taking 12–24 months.
- Patellar subluxation is not uncommon, detected when the knee is in full extension. Displacing the patella laterally results in the patient grabbing the examiner's hand (apprehension sign).
- Painful ankle may be due to sport injury (the most common cause) or referred pain from avascular necrosis of the navicular bone (Köhler's disease) or the metatarsal head (Freiberg's disease).
- Although persistent arthralgia without evidence of arthritis is uncommon in JIA, arthralgia lasting several weeks may occur in the pre-arthritic stage of the disease.

Red Flags

- Knee joint pain may be a referred pain originating from a diseased hip, such as transient synovitis. The knee joint is more superficial than the hip and both share common nerve branches.
- Arthralgia due to a malignancy is typically disproportionally constant and severe compared to the clinical findings. FBC may reveal low Hb and platelets and diagnostic peripheral blood smear (for leukaemia).
- Early diagnosis of leukaemia is important. The use of steroids and immunosuppressants without excluding haematological malignancy is likely to mask and delay the diagnosis.
- Remember that the diagnosis of juvenile idiopathic arthritis should only be made if there is evidence of arthritis (not arthralgia) persistent for more than 6 weeks and if other diagnoses have been excluded.

FURTHER READING

Yilmaz AE, Atalar H, Tag T et al. Knee joint pain may be an indication for a hip joint problem in children: A case report. *Malays J Med Sci* 2011;18(1):79–82.

Zombori L, Kovacs G, Csoka M et al. Rheumatic symptoms in childhood leukaemia and lymphoma – A ten-year retrospective study. *Pediatr Rheumatol Online J* 2013;11:20.

ARTHRITIS (SWOLLEN JOINTS)

Clinical Overview

A detailed discussion on arthritis, which comprises more than 100 different diseases, is beyond the scope of this book. In short, arthritis may be monoarthritis, oligoarthritis (less than five joints) or polyarthritis (five or more joints). The main causes of oligoarthritis are trauma, septic arthritis, JIA, reactive arthritis (ReA), Lyme disease, transient synovitis, neoplastic arthritis and tuberculosis (TB) arthritis. Causes of polyarthritis include JIA, rheumatic fever (RF), and vasculitis. JIA and ReA are forms of autoimmune arthritis. ReA develops in response to an infection, occurring 1–3 weeks elsewhere in the body, most commonly following a viral or intestinal infection (*Campylobacter, Salmonella* or *Yersinia*). JIA is classified into systemic onset (associated with high remittent fever, rash, generalised lymphadenopathy, hepatosplenomegaly and serositis), oligoarthritis and polyarthritis.

Possible Diagnoses

Infants	Children
Common	
Post-infectious arthritis	Post-infectious arthritis (reactive, synovitis)
Septic arthritis	JIA
Collagen disease	Transient synovitis (TS)
JIA	Vasculitis (e.g. Henoch–Schönlein disease)
Vasculitis	Septic arthritis (SA)
Rare	
	Familial Mediterranean fever
	Trauma
	Rheumatic fever
	Arthritis of inflammatory bowel disease
	Lyme disease
	Neoplastic arthritis (leukaemia, lymphoma)
	TB arthritis
	Psoriatic arthritis
	Behçet's disease
	Reactive arthritis

Differential Diagnosis at a Glance

	Post-Infectious	JIA	Transient Synovitis	Vasculitis	SA
Fever >39.0°C	Possible	Possible	No	Possible	Yes
Monoarthritis	Possible	Possible	Yes	No	Yes
Persistent more than 6 weeks	No	Yes	No	No	No
Associated skin rash	Possible	Possible	No	Yes	No
High anti-nuclear antibodies (ANAs)	Possible	Possible	No	No	No

Recommended Investigations

*** FBC: erythrocyte sedimentation rate (ESR), WBC, and platelets raised in many rheumatic diseases, including JIA

*** Auto-antibodies, such as ANAs: positive in the majority of JIA

*** Rheumatoid factor, particularly in cases of polyarthritis JIA

*** Magnetic resonance imaging (MRI) is the only tool with the ability to assess disease activity in the joints of JIA

*** Bone marrow aspiration: positive in early stage of septic arthritis (SA) or transient synovitis

** Bone scan, X-ray and MRI: diagnostic in suspected cases of neoplastic arthritis

** Children with juvenile arthritis should be referred for an ophthalmological evaluation

Top Tips

- When a child presents with arthritis, the first question is as follows: is it monoarthritis, oligoarthritis or polyarthritis? That alone can restrict the differential diagnosis.
- Transient synovitis is diagnosed by a mild or no fever, history of a viral upper respiratory tract infection and one hip being affected. Child appears well – limping but still walking. WBC, CRP and ESR are usually normal; WBC count in the joint fluid is <50,000 cells/mm. It is self-limiting, usually lasting 1–3 weeks.
- Systemic onset JIA can be diagnosed by the intermittent high fever, often hectic, with a daily rise in the evening, then falling to normal in the morning. The pattern may become double quotidian. Fever is often associated with the occurrence of rash, lymphadenopathy and splenomegaly.
- SA, usually monoarthritis, is characterised by high fever >39.5°C, severe pain, restricted range of joint movement and refusal to walk. It is defined as positive joint fluid culture for bacteria and/or WBC count in the joint fluid of >50,000 cells/mm, mainly polymorphonuclear cells.
- RF is characterised by migratory arthritis, occurring 2–3 weeks following an untreated group A ß-haemolytic streptococcal pharyngitis. Diagnosis is established by Jones criteria.
- ANAs are specific for nuclear constituents. These are important arthritis tests: they are positive in nearly 100% in mixed connective tissue disease, in over 95% in SLE and in about 50% in JIA.

Red Flags

- Uveitis may be the initial presentation of JIA, particularly with oligoarthritis. One-third of children develop unilateral (even bilateral) loss of visual acuity. Regular eye checks are essential.
- Neoplastic arthritis should always be borne in mind. Diagnostic clues include the presence of lymphadenopathy, hepatosplenomegaly, anaemia, thrombocytopenia, or blast cells on the peripheral blood smear; pyrexia is usually mild or absent. Bone marrow aspiration is diagnostic.
- Temporomandibular arthritis in JIA is challenging to evaluate because of the absence of joint swelling. If untreated early, devastating effects occur in its form and function.
- In TB arthritis there is typically a lack of response to treatment with antibiotics, non-steroidal anti-inflammatory drugs or intraocular steroids. Diagnosis is by positive Mantoux test, with possible TB lesions in a chest X-ray and synovial biopsy.

FURTHER READING

Barut K, Adrovic A, Sahin S et al. Juvenile idiopathic arthritis. *Balkan Med J* 2017;34(2):90–101.

Stoll M, Kau CH, Waite PD et al. Temporomandibular joint arthritis in juvenile idiopathic arthritis, now what? *Pediatr Rheumatol Online J* 2018;16:32.

BACK PAIN

Clinical Overview

Back pain is a common complaint in adults, but it often begins in children and adolescents. It is one of the most reported health problems worldwide and a leading cause of disability, activity limitation and school absences. Low back pain is the most common type of back pain and is defined as pain limited to the region between the lower margins of the 12th rib and the gluteal folds, with or without referred leg pain. The majority of causes of back pain have an underlying musculoskeletal or biochemical origin, such as trauma, muscle strain or infectious and inflammatory diseases. Acute onset of pain is suggestive of trauma or infection, while insidious onset may suggest inflammatory or neoplastic aetiology. Localised back pain may suggest stress fracture, while non-localised pain is often secondary to muscular or inflammatory cause. Pyelonephritis is an important cause of back pain.

Possible Diagnoses

Infants	Children
Common	
	Trauma
	Infection (e.g. pyogenic, TB)
	Spondylolysis/spondylolisthesis
	Neuropathic
	Neoplasms
	Scheuermann's disease
Rare	
	Sacroiliitis
	Ankylosing spondylitis

Differential Diagnosis at a Glance

	Trauma	Infection	Spondylolysis	Neuropathic	Neoplasms
Acute onset	Yes	Yes	No	Possible	No
Fever	No	Yes	No	No	Possible
Burning, pins and needles	No	No	No	Yes	Possible
High WBC, CRP	No	Yes	No	No	Possible
Diagnostic MRI	Possible	Possible	Yes	Yes	Yes

Recommended Investigations

*** FBC, with ESR and/or CRP for inflammatory spinal diseases
*** Rheumatoid factor, HLA-B27 in suspected cases of ankylosing spondylitis
*** MRI is the only tool with the ability to assess disease activity in the joints of those with JIA
*** Children with suspected spinal cord lesions should undergo spine MRI with and without contrast

Top Tips

- Neuropathic back pain refers to pain arising from injury or disease directly affecting the nerve roots that innervate the spine and legs. Cardinal symptoms include spontaneous pain (e.g. shooting or electric shock-like), abnormal response to non-painful stimuli (e.g. light touch), abnormal thermal sensation (burning or ice-cold) and pricking pins and needles sensation.
- Spondylolysis is a unilateral fracture and spondylolisthesis is a bilateral fracture of the pars inter-articularis. Both may occur as congenital spinal abnormality or commonly resulting from back hyperextension following athletic injury (football, gymnastics or swimming) with anterior displacement of the vertebral body on X-ray.
- Scheuermann's disease is characterised by increasing thoracic or thoraco-lumbar kyphosis with tightness of the hamstrings and iliopsoas muscles. Diagnosis is a spinal X-ray showing anterior wedging greater than five degrees of three or more consecutive vertebrae.

Red Flags

- A schoolbag that exceeds 10% of body weight can lead to back pain and later becomes chronic.
- Back pain in association with fever and focal tenderness raises the possibility of serious pathology.
- Persistent and localised back pain that is worse at night may suggest either a benign cause (e.g. osteoid osteoma or bone cyst) or a malignant neoplasm (e.g. Ewing's sarcoma, lymphoma or neuroblastoma).
- Be aware of the high incidence of uveitis in suspected cases of ankylosing spondylitis.

FURTHER READING

Calvo-Munoz I, Gomez-Conesa A, Sanchez-Meca J. Prevalence of low back pain in children and adolescents: A meta-analysis. *BMC Pediatr* 2013;13:14.

Taxter AJ, Chauvin NA, Weiss PF. Diagnosis and treatment of low back pain in children and adolescents. *Phys Sportmed* 2014;42(1):94–104.

MYALGIA (PAINFUL MUSCLES)

Clinical Overview

Acute muscle pain (myalgia) is a common complaint occurring in association with minor trauma, muscle overuse and viral infections. It is not due to systemic or local spread of the microorganisms, but rather due to interleukin-1 effect, which induces protein breakdown (proteolysis). Myalgia can be due to benign causes, such as musculoskeletal injury (sprains, strains, contusions or overuse) or musculoskeletal pain syndrome (MSPS), or to more serious conditions, such as myopathies (e.g. dermatomyositis or polymyositis), metabolic disorders (glycogen storage disease) or muscular dystrophies (e.g. dystrophinopathies including Duchenne muscular dystrophy). Occasionally, myalgia can be recurrent (e.g. familial Mediterranean fever) or chronic (e.g. chronic musculoskeletal pain).

Possible Diagnoses

Infants	Children
Common	
Birth injury (muscle pulling or fracture)	Febrile illness (e.g. viral myositis)
Any febrile illness	MSPS
Child abuse	Familial Mediterranean fever (FMF)
Trauma	CTD
Connective tissue disease (CTD)	Chronic fatigue syndrome (CFS)
Rare	
Metabolic (fatty acids oxidation defect)	Child abuse
Scurvy	Trauma
	Fibromyalgia
	Infections (e.g. influenza b, Lyme disease, Dengue, brucellosis)
	Acute polyneuropathy
	Mitochondrial disease
	Drugs (statins or carbimazole)
	Porphyria
	Bornholm disease
	Trichinosis
	Polymyalgia rheumatica
	Cutaneous vasculitis
	Wegener's granulomatosis
	Glycogen storage disease

Differential Diagnosis at a Glance

	Febrile illness	MSPS	FMF	CTD	CFS
Diffuse	Yes	No	Yes	Possible	Yes
Fever	Yes	No	Yes	Possible	Possible
Associated fatigue	Possible	Possible	Possible	Possible	Yes
Mainly 1–3 years	Yes	Possible	No	Possible	No
Abnormal WBC, CRP	Possible	No	Possible	Yes	No

Recommended Investigations

*** Urine: proteinuria in SLE; urine for porphyrins, porphyria and rhabdomyolysis
*** FBC may be helpful in showing leucopenia, thrombocytopenia and anaemia in SLE
*** CRP (or ESR) is helpful for bacterial infections, CTD, dermatomyositis and FMF
*** Auto-antibodies such as ANA are helpful in CTD
*** For trichinosis, serological studies and muscle biopsy (showing larvae) confirm the diagnosis
*** Ultrasound scan and/or MRI is helpful in some inflammatory conditions
*** Serological and microbiological studies in children with suspected infection-related myalgia

Top Tips

- Not all muscle diseases produce pain; muscle diseases not associated with myalgia include muscular dystrophy and spinal muscular atrophies.
- Acute myositis usually follows recovery from a viral illness. Children present with symmetrical leg pain and refusal to walk. The condition is usually benign and self-limiting within a few days.
- Chronic musculoskeletal pain is usually caused by non-inflammatory conditions such as joint hypermobility. Affected pre-pubertal children recover more rapidly than post-pubertal.
- Diagnostic criteria for FMF are recurring episodes of fever; pain in the abdomen (peritonitis), chest (pleuritis) or joints (arthritis); and muscles (myalgia).
- Clinicians should be aware that there are overlapping symptoms among MSPS, fibromyalgia, CFS and reflex sympathetic dystrophy.
- Fibromyalgia is associated with widespread pain and stiffness in the muscles, sleep disturbance, school absence and fatigue. The condition may need to be differentiated from CFS.

Red Flags

- In any child with unexplained muscle pain, child abuse should be considered among the differential diagnoses. Skeletal survey may be needed to confirm it.
- Occasionally a case of acute viral myositis may develop rhabdomyolysis requiring dialysis.
- Acute viral myositis is often mistaken for neurological illness such as Guillain–Barré syndrome or autoimmune disease leading to unnecessary investigation.
- A child with acute muscular weakness affecting the limb girdle muscles should be suspected of having dermatomyositis until proven otherwise. A peri-orbital rash is an important clue.
- Myalgia can be the presenting symptom of some serious diseases including bone tumours.
- Although trichinosis is uncommon in children in this country, it is common worldwide (e.g. USA, less common nowadays). Children present with localised myalgia and fever. Eosinophilia is present in blood. A clue is ingestion of raw or undercooked pork meat.

FURTHER READING

Magee H, Goldman RD. Viral myositis in children. *Can Family Physician* 2017;63(5):365–368.

PAINFUL ARM

Clinical Overview

In children, arm pain usually results from musculoskeletal injuries (sprain, strain, contusion, dislocation and fracture). In the absence of dislocation or fracture, a MSPS or childhood fibromyalgia can be considered. Both are diagnoses of exclusion. The pain may affect part of the arm, the whole upper arm or the forearm, occurring suddenly or gradually, constantly or intermittently and often associated with a burning or numbing sensation. If there is a history suggestive of injury (e.g. sport activity), the diagnosis is evident. A moderate to severe injury is likely to be followed by an inflammatory response that manifests as pain, spasm, reduced arm movement and redness and swelling. Less common causes of arm pain include neurovascular, cardiovascular disorders and referred pain from another area such as the neck, chest or abdomen.

Possible Diagnoses

Infants	Children
Common	
Birth injury	MSPS
Pulled elbow (nursemaid's elbow)	Dislocation, fracture (including nursemaid's elbow)
Myalgia (e.g. viral infection)	Myalgia (e.g. viral infection)
Child abuse	Tendonitis and tenosynovitis
Infection (osteomyelitis)	Arthritis
Rare	
Child abuse	Child abuse
Bone tumour	CFS
Scurvy	Fibromyalgia
Arthritis	Complex regional pain syndrome
	Cervical nerve root compression
	Malignancy (bone tumour)
	Osteomyelitis
	Neuritis (neuropathy), compartment syndrome
	Scurvy
	Fabry's disease (lysosomal disease with neuropathy)
	Raynaud's phenomenon

Differential Diagnosis at a Glance

	MSPS	Dislocation/ Fracture	Myalgia	Tendonitis	Arthritis
Non-arthritic pain	Yes	No	Yes	Possible	No
Usually mild	Possible	No	Yes	Possible	No
Associated swelling/tender	Yes	Possible	No	Yes	Yes
Fever	No	No	Possible	No	Yes
Normal laboratory WBC, CRP	Yes	Yes	Possible	Yes	No

Recommended Investigations

*** High FBC and CRP will support bacterial infection or arthritis
** Autoantibody screen is useful in case of Raynaud's phenomenon
*** X-ray of the arm to exclude fracture or dislocation
*** Spinal X-ray is indicated if spinal lesions are suspected
** Bone scan in case of suspected osteomyelitis or malignancy

Top Tips

- Pain in the elbow may be caused by nursemaid's elbow (pulling hard on the child's hand or wrist).
- MSPS is a diagnosis of exclusion. Pain may be persistent, localised or diffuse, characteristically increasing over time, and associated with muscle tenderness, allodynia (pain resulting from stimulation such as light touch of the skin) and incongruent effect (inappropriate effect with the situation, with common associated anxiety and depression). If affects often pre- to adolescent girls.
- Childhood fibromyalgia is characterised by generalised musculoskeletal pain at several sites (at least four), with typical tenderness at several points, lasting more than 3 months.
- Fibromyalgia may be associated with irritable bowel syndrome (incidence around 50%), migraine or tension headaches (incidence around 50%) or temporomandibular joint dysfunction.
- Fibromyalgia and complex regional pain syndrome are variant manifestations of MSPS. Although symptoms often overlap with MSPS, they tend to be prolonged and recurrent.
- Although growing pain affects the lower extremities more often than the upper extremities, arms may be involved. Remember its criteria: pain is episodic, typically nocturnal, non-articular, with no daytime disability and continues for months.
- Compartment syndrome is rare in children, affecting circulation and function due to increased pressure in a confined space, causing severe pain to be felt with passive muscle stretching.

Red Flags

- The presence of paraesthesiae, such as numbness, suggests a neurological condition, e.g. neuritis or nerve trapping. Beware that children may interpret paraesthesiae and muscle weakness as pain. Careful history taking and physical examination are essential.
- The possibility of child abuse, Munchausen's syndrome by proxy and school phobia should always be considered in the differential diagnosis for a young child with unexplained pain.
- In any child with a trauma, peripheral pulses and capillary refill time must be checked.
- Despite the overlap of symptoms, MSPS, fibromyalgia and CFS must be differentiated. MSPS and fibromyalgia are associated with pain; in CFS the striking symptom is fatigue.
- Beware that Raynaud's phenomenon can present with swelling and pain of the fingers and forearm. If this phenomenon worsens over time, autoimmune diseases such as dermatomyositis, systemic scleroderma or SLE could be the underlying cause.

FURTHER READING

Gmuca S, Sherry DD. Fibromyalgia: Treating pain in the juvenile patient. *Pediatr Drugs* 2017;19(4):325–338.

PAINFUL LEG AND LIMPING

Clinical Overview

Pain in the leg is common and caused by musculoskeletal disorders, mainly as a result of trauma, developmental, infectious and rheumatological and neoplastical disorders. Painful limping is the usual presentation. The majority of musculoskeletal causes are benign, self-limiting and often trauma related. To facilitate an easy approach, age-related disorders are classified in three groups: *infant-toddler group (1–3 years)*: non-specific muscular pain, poor-fitting shoes, trauma, congenital hip dislocation (CDH) (unnoticed at birth), transient synovitis, avascular necrosis, septic arthritis, JIA, mild CP, or tumours. *School-age group (4–10 years)*: non-specific muscular pain, growing pain, Perthes' disease. *Adolescent age (11–15 years)*: osteochondritis, slipped capital femoral epiphysis (SCFE), osteochondritis dissecans and idiopathic adolescent knee pain syndrome. The key to an accurate diagnosis is careful history taking, thorough physical and neurological examination and appropriate radiological and laboratory investigations.

Possible Diagnoses

Infants	Children
Common	
Congenital hip dislocation	Trauma (minor muscle strains/sprains/overuse)
Fracture	Growing pain
Child abuse	Transient synovitis
Infection (e.g. septic arthritis)	Avascular necrosis (e.g. Perthes' disease, SCFE)
Arthritis/arthralgia	Arthralgia/arthritis
Rare	
Osteochondritis in syphilis	Septic arthritis
Congenital hip dislocation	Discoid meniscus
Scurvy	Cerebral palsy (e.g. hemiplegia)
	Limb length discrepancy (e.g. CDH)
	Malignancy (leukaemia [acute lymphoblastic leukemia, ALL], osteoma)
	Duchenne muscular dystrophy (DMD)
	Psychiatric diseases (e.g. conversion disorder)
	SCA
	Congenital hip dislocation (unnoticed at birth)
	Drugs (steroids)
	Complex regional pain syndrome
	Ankylosing spondylitis

Differential Diagnosis at a Glance

	Trauma	Growing Pain	Transient Synovitis	Avascular Necrosis	Arthralgia/ Arthritis
MS tenderness	Yes	No	Possible	Yes	Yes
Fever	No	No	Possible	No	Possible
Limping	Possible	No	Yes	Yes	Yes
Nocturnal pain	Possible	Yes	No	No	No
Diagnosis by X-ray	No	No	No	Yes	No

Recommended Investigations

*** FBC and CRP for infectious diseases (e.g. osteomyelitis or arthritis)
*** Rheumatoid factor, ANAs, human leukocyte antigen B27 for rheumatological cases
*** CPK, serum transaminases for muscular diseases
*** TFTs and growth hormone level in pre-pubertal children with SCFE
*** X-ray of the leg can diagnose many disorders, e.g. tumour or avascular necrosis
** MRI and bone scan are indicated by the result of the X-ray

Top Tips

- Before diagnosing a disease in a child with leg pain and limping, examine the shoes for poor fit or any foreign body such as a nail. These are common causes.
- The history of growing pain is diagnostic: non-articular pain occurring at night for at least 6 months and normal physical examination.
- Limping may be due to discrepancy of the leg length: measurement of the leg is performed by a tape measure of the distance between anterior iliac spine and the medial malleolus.
- CDH may pass unnoticed at birth and presentation is with limping. If CDH is unilateral, the affected limb is shortened by at least 2 cm (significant). If bilateral, gait resembles duck walk due to increased lumbar lordosis.
- In a child with preceding upper respiratory tract infection who is afebrile with sudden limping, transient synovitis is very likely. Laboratory and radiological investigations are usually normal.
- Although X-rays of the leg are often requested for suspected cases of avascular necrosis (osteochondrosis), a more important reason is to exclude other lesions such as tumour.
- Long-term use of steroids can cause osteoporosis, fractures and avascular necrosis.

Red Flags

- Beware that children older than 10 years with Perthes' disease will almost certainly develop degenerative arthritis later on.
- Any boy with a delayed walking age of 18 months and DMD should be excluded by checking the serum CPK. Children present with repeated stumbling and falls and difficulty climbing upstairs.
- When the knee is examined, patello-femoral crepitations may be elicited. This is common in normal individuals and does not indicate a knee disease.
- Remember that imaging of the bone is normal in the early stages of Perthes' disease; the 'crescent sign' in a frog lateral position is the earliest possible radiological sign.
- Many children with hip diseases present with knee pain. Pain in Perthes' disease typically manifests in the groin and thigh, radiating to the knee. Examination of all joints is essential.
- In a young child with an unexplained pain, child abuse should not be forgotten in the differential diagnosis. Examine the skin carefully for relevant bruises; skeletal survey may be required.
- SCFE is the most common hip disorder in adolescence. If it occurs pre-pubertally, an endocrine cause such as hypothyroidism or growth hormone deficiency may be the underlying pathology.
- In children with ALL, more than 50% present with bone involvement with limping and pain typically in the morning, mainly in the lower extremities.

FURTHER READING

Santili C, Junior W, Golano EO et al. Limping in children. *Rev Bras Orthop* 2009;44(4):290–294.
Tragiannidis A, Vasileiou E, Papageoiou M et al. Bone involvement at diagnosis as a predictive factor in children with acute lymphoblastic leukemia. *Hippokrata* 2016;20(3):227–230.

INDEX

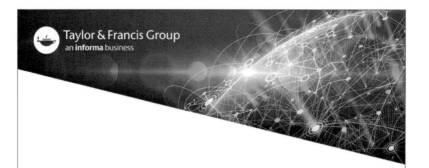